Testosterone revolution

Testosterone revolution

Rediscover Your Energy and Overcome the Symptoms of Male Menopause

MALCOLM CARRUTHERS
MD,FRCPATH,MRCGP

Thorsons

To the father—in his many forms

Thorsons
An Imprint of HarperCollins*Publishers*
77–85 Fulham Palace Road
Hammersmith, London W6 8JB

The Thorsons website address is:
www.thorsons.com

Thorsons is a trademark of
HarperCollins *Publishers* Limited

Originally published in hardback by HarperCollins as *Male Menopause* in 1996
This edition published by Thorsons 2001

10 9 8 7 6 5 4 3 2 1

© Malcolm Carruthers 1996, 2001

Malcolm Carruthers asserts the moral right to
be identified as the author of this work.

A catalogue record for this book
is available from the British Library

ISBN 0 00 712275 6

Printed and bound in Great Britain by
Creative Print and Design Wales, Ebbw Vale

Contents

Foreword

I joined the Men's Health Movement on November 21, 1969 with the birth of my first son. I vowed to be a different kind of father than the one I had been raised with and to help bring about a world where both males and females would be healthy, free and equal.

Six years earlier Betty Friedan had helped to launch the modern feminist movement with the publication of her book, *The Feminine Mystique*. There was the recognition that gender played a significant role in our health and well-being and many women's health programs were initiated over the next ten years. It seemed clear that there was a need for parallel programs for men.

This seemed to be happening. In 1973 Martha Weinman Lear wrote an article for the *New York Times Magazine*, asking, 'Is There a Male Menopause?' Warren Farrell titled the first chapter of his 1974 book, *The Liberated Man*, 'Women's Liberation and the Masculine Mystique: The Neglected Connection.' However, men's health didn't catch on like women's health did.

Although there were a few of us who tried to keep the men's health movement going, over the years it lost steam. The women's movement continued to grow and prosper. As we moved into the 1980s men seemed more interested in wealth than in health. In the USA, gender health became synonymous with women's health.

When I began doing research for my book, *Male Menopause*, I found little information in America. I found, however, that a lot had been going on outside the USA and one of the leading clinicians was Dr Malcolm Carruthers. In over twenty years of research he was able to answer Lear's question, 'Is There a Male Menopause?' with an emphatic, 'Yes!' His ongoing research on testosterone replacement therapy is providing information that will help all men live long and well. Dr Carruthers is now bringing the results of his own wide-ranging research, and the research of the world-health community, to us.

I believe we are primed and ready for Dr Carruthers' critically important message. We are older and wiser. We want gender medicine to include *both* genders. This need is reflected in a resolution before

Congress to form the Office of Men's Health that would parallel the already well-established Office of Women's Health.

There are many reasons I am excited to be recommending this book to you. It contains the most authoritative information you will find anywhere. You will learn specific things you can do to insure that your sex life not only won't decline, but can also improve with age. You will find out how to protect your heart and your bones, and ways to keep from getting a potbelly. It is fun and enjoyable to read. You'll find yourself underlining page after page.

There are a number of books available on men's health and a few on the importance of testosterone in a man's life. However, no other book explores the subject matter from such a balanced perspective. Although Dr Carruthers recognizes the critical value of testosterone, he also knows the importance of physical, psychological, interpersonal, social, and spiritual aspects of men's health.

Reading Dr Carruthers' book is like talking to the physician most of us wish we had – someone who is accessible, knowledgeable, compassionate, caring and who doesn't take life too seriously. This is a rare book written by a wise healer. It is a book that will change your life for the better. Jump in and enjoy. You'll be glad you did.

Jed Diamond
Director of MenAlive
Author, *Male Menopause and Surviving Male Menopause: A Guide For Women and Men*

Acknowledgements

Help is gratefully acknowledged in three areas:

In the production of this book, Wanda Whiteley initiated it, and Samantha Grant, assistant health editor, gently persevered in its evolution and completion. The whole Thorsons publishing team has been a pleasure to work with throughout.

The medical research on which this work is based was supported partly by grants from the European Organization for the Control of Circulatory Diseases (EOCCD) and the Sophus Jacobsen og hustru Astrid Jacobsen's Fond and LBK Foundation in Copenhagen, Denmark, as well as Drs Jens Moller and Michael Hansen, previous and current presidents of these organizations.

The author also wishes to thank Dr Jamie Zadeh, Doreen Jackson and Graham Carter of the Department of Endocrinology at the Charing Cross Hospital London, where the pathology tests were initially performed; subsequently the laboratory tests were carried out at Unilabs, and by Quest Diagnostic Laboratories in the UK, to which I am particularly grateful for making tests also available in the USA.

I am also indebted for much wise advice and encouragement from Professor Vivian James of the Department of Steroid Endocrinology, St Mary's Hospital, London; Dr Neil O'Donoghue of the Institute of Urology, London, and Col. Douglas W. Soderdahl FACS, Chief of Urology, the Honolulu Medical Group, for constructive advice and criticism.

In Australia, Linda Byart, Dr Adrian Zentner, and their other colleagues at the Wellmen Centers in Perth and throughout the country have been towers of strength in the ongoing fight for the right of men to have TRT.

More recently, Dr Bruce Wilkin of Ely, Nevada has been endlessly kind, both in giving me books on the history of testosterone and 'High-T' men, supporting the AndroScreen web site and as host during my visit to an awe-inspiring part of the USA. Similarly, Dr Pat Puglio, her daughter Cindy and all the staff of the Broda O. Barnes Foundation in Stamford, Connecticut, were the kindest of conference organizers and their friendship helped me to establish a bridgehead for the testosterone revolution in America. Also, Jed Diamond, both by his writing and by holding a series of conferences on 'Male Menopause,' sponsored by his MenAlive health center in San Francisco, has been most helpful and supportive of the men's movement, of which my work is a part.

I would also like to thank my colleagues Dr Duncan Gould, Dr John Tomlinson, Dr Pierre Bouloux and Mr Farook Al-Azzawi, fellow members of the committee of The Andropause Society for their help in fermenting the world-wide 'Testosterone Revolution.'

Mr Hugh Welford, webmaster extraordinary, who created brilliant and elegant computer programs to handle the mass of data from patients in the London Clinic and all over the world, to the AndroScreen and Andropause Society web sites, has been my best man in every sense of the term.

My wife Jean has also been endlessly loving, kind and supportive throughout the 20 years' drama of the revolution, taking part in most of the battles leading up to it, and helping me survive at every level. An important part of this has been her work as Secretary of the Andropause Society, helping this charity into existence, as she did with The Autogenic Society 20 years ago.

Also on the personal level, my brother Dr Barry Carruthers influenced my choice of career and sparked my interest in andrology. Dr Janet Carruthers gave me the opportunity to experience the joys of fatherhood, as did my three sons Ian, Andrew and Robert, who gave helpful comments on earlier versions of this book.

Finally, my thanks are due to many of my patients whose experiences are recorded here, particularly those who were brave and supportive enough to 'stand up and be counted' in the newspapers, radio and television. Special thanks are due to Bernard Collen and his wife Michele, to James Savin, Robert Bain and Spencer Churchill. Now that 'Male Menopause' or 'Andropause' is finally becoming accepted as a biological fact of life for some men, and male HRT is becoming a standard method of treatment and an accepted part of preventive medicine, these people deserve to be recognized as true heroes of the 'Testosterone Revolution.'

The Male Menopause Mystery

What is the mystery of male menopause? It is the mystery of why the vitality and virility of millions of men disappears in middle age or later. It is the mystery of why most people and their doctors deny, ignore or unquestioningly accept this disappearance – and of why no attempt is made to investigate this loss or try to reclaim it, despite evidence that this is often possible.

As in most detective stories, the answer lies in asking the right questions and hopefully finding the right answers, piecing together the jigsaw puzzle until the picture jumps out at you. Many investigators have already searched the area for many years without stumbling on the truth. Let's start with a few questions and think about the clues we might follow up to find the answers.

What is missing?

The typical story is of a man in middle age who gradually loses his drive, strength, energy and enthusiasm for life and love. Action man has become inaction man. An all-pervasive mental and physical tiredness descends on him, often for no apparent reason. He changes from being a positive, bullish, outgoing person who is good to be around to a negative, pessimistic, depressed grouch who is increasingly difficult to live or work with. At work he is seen to have lost his edge and no amount of encouragement or urging will improve his performance. At home, family relations become increasingly strained, and social life dwindles. His sexual life is usually a disaster area, with loss of libido and intermittent failure to achieve an erection leading to performance anxiety and eventually complete impotence. This creates a downward spiral of failing function in the bedroom and boardroom.

When, after ignoring or denying his condition for months or even years, the quietly desperate man goes to a doctor, all he is told is, 'So you feel tired, dispirited, exhausted and your sex life is nonexistent? It's your age. I feel like that, too. What do you expect? So your wife had the same symptoms when she went through menopause and got hormones from her gynecologist which revitalized her so much that you can't keep up? That doesn't apply to *you* – there's no such thing as male menopause or male hormone replacement therapy. Just forget it and take these antidepressants – they'll make us both feel better.'

Why the denial?

Why do neither doctors nor patients recognize male menopause as a real medical condition worthy of being diagnosed and treated? Because, even if dignified with the medical title of 'andropause,' as it is known in Europe, it is still an unacceptable threat to their macho self-image. It is the joke illness attributed to any middle-aged male character in a sitcom who behaves in an unexpected or irrational fashion. Men see it as the end of their lives as potent males, as leaders and as lovers.

While female menopause usually happens in the limited age range of 45–55, the symptoms in men can start any time from 30 onward, though they too tend to peak at 50. Interestingly, 50, the 'Big Five-O,' appears to be a watershed in the lives of both men and women. Yet this should be simply half time in the game of life, the goal being 100 years of activity and enjoyment! Why do men put up with losing so much so young?

Gail Sheehy, an American author who has written a fascinating book on male and female life cycles, *New Passages*,[1] describes male menopause as the 'unspeakable passage.'[2] While women are willing to discuss their menopause with each other and with their medical advisers, men are remarkably reluctant to turn to either unless they are desperate. In fact they are likely to get very angry with anyone, even their nearest and dearest, who might suggest that they need any treatment. If cancer is the unmentionable 'Big C,' male menopause is the even more unspeakable 'Big M.'

Logically, there should be no shame attached to this condition. Indeed, as we shall see later, it is often the result of living life to the fullest which causes it. The most macho of males can suffer from it. But even men who have greatly improved with testosterone treatment will rarely go public for fear of being thought weak or being ridiculed by their friends or relatives. Fortunately there is an increasing number of men who are willing to stand up and be counted, and they greatly help getting the condition and its treatment recognized by doing so.

Why has testosterone had such a bad press?

Another problem is the public perception of testosterone as the hormone responsible for undesirable male traits such as aggression and hypersexuality. So surely testosterone replacement therapy (TRT) will 'bring out the beast?' The fear, which in practice is unfounded, of becoming a rapacious monster like Jack Nicholson in the film 'Wolf,' holds back from treatment many menopausal men who, unlike him, cannot claim to have 'retained my testosterone longer than most males.'

Also, reports of abuse of anabolic steroids by athletes and bodybuilders, together with deliberately exaggerated horror stories of the physical and psychological dangers of the drugs, have appeared in the newspapers increasingly frequently over the last 20 years.[3,4] As testosterone is the basic compound from which all other anabolic steroids are derived, it has suffered a very bad press by association.

Why isn't biotechnology coming up with the answers?

Linked to these factors is the extreme reluctance of most drug firms to consider funding research about testosterone replacement therapy for men, even though estrogen replacement therapy for women is a rapidly expanding market, already estimated to be worth over £50 million annually world-wide.

The product licenses have expired on existing testosterone preparations, many which have proven safe and successful for up to 50 years, so that anyone can make them but with smaller profit margins. There is also the risk of litigation by patients suffering side effects. These sex hormones just aren't sexy any more. Even so, common sense would suggest that the market is huge for long-acting forms that are easier to take. This would make TRT more popular, cheaper and more available. Yet most doctors interested in developing new forms of testosterone treatment have faced the extreme apathy or even antipathy of pharmaceutical companies.

Why shouldn't we just grow old 'gracefully'?

Many doctors, politicians and economists argue that no country can afford the cost of 'his and hers HRT.' Who wants to keep an increasing number of 'golden oldies' going anyway? It isn't natural.

Yet women over the last 30 years or more have fought successfully to maintain their hormonal status into later life, with all the consequent medical benefits. Supporters of 'men's lib' would say that they have in this respect been sadly neglected; they live seven or eight years less than women, and it's time they had a chance to catch up in the health stakes.

There are also many good reasons for regarding 'his and hers HRT' as an important part of the preventive medicine of the future, helping both sexes to prolong an active and enjoyable life. It adds life to years as well as years to life. Health economic theorists have also pointed out the substantial savings to be made by shortening the terminal period of disability and incapacity, which would give many people a happier ending to life.[5]

Of course, something will fail at some time in our body's systems, but shouldn't we at least be looking at every reasonable option for staying as mentally and physically active as we can, for as long as possible? The benefits have to be weighed against costs and dangers, but doctors should be continually assessing the evidence for and against each treatment and offering it to patients to decide for themselves.

Given the wide range of benefits to psyche, soma and sexuality that hormone therapy provides, increasing numbers of people view it as modern science giving nature a helping hand.

Why doesn't medical science recognize the problem?

The reasons for this are many, and illustrate very well how ideas come into and go out of fashion and style.

Medical theory does not advance in a straight line, but in a series of loops. Essentially scientists come across facts from which they make up a theory which is then taught to students and other doctors. The theory is then 'in.' Taking that as their starting point, the scientists trudge around the loop, gathering more facts, until they find some which seem to contradict the original theory. Then the theory is 'out.' Never mind, change the teaching, change the textbooks and go on, regardless.

Then the scientists rediscover some of the ideas of those who originally thought up the theory which lead right back to the starting point. To avoid the worrying realization that they've just walked in a complete circle, they add a few new facts to prove it right after all. The old theory is dusted off, decorated with a glamorous statistical wig to cover a few bald facts, given some reference make-up, and then brought right back 'in' again.

In case you think I exaggerate a little, let me give you a brief account of the curious history of theories about whether male menopause is a real or imaginary condition.

Ideas about what gives a man both vitality and virility, and why these qualities vary from person to person and at different stages in life, are as old as recorded history. Certainly, at the end of the eighteenth century the concept of male menopause or 'decline' as it was then called, was definitely 'in.' A Dr Hooper, living in London, wrote in his *Medical Dictionary*, 'Decline in men is a real malady and not a natural or constitutional decay, as is perfectly obvious from recovery.'[5] He had observed that men could sometimes make a remarkable recovery when their businesses prospered or a new woman came into their lives.[6]

About 100 years later attempts were made to rejuvenate older men by injecting testicular extracts and even whole testes from different species. In general, these 'monkey gland' treatments, as they became known, got a bad name because they were usually ineffective and were largely practiced by quacks out to make a fast buck out of old bucks. These practices discredited the idea of male menopause and its treatment, which then went 'out,' and left a stain upon the good name of testosterone which persists to this day.

It was only when testosterone was isolated and then synthesized in industrial quantities from 1935 onward that effective replacement therapy with this hormone became possible. This brought theories about male menopause or 'male climacteric' – another medical term for decline – back into favor again, and for a while everything was clear and scientifically respectable.[7]

Excellent articles and books appeared in the medical literature of the 1940s, accurately documenting the symptoms of male menopause and noting how similar they were to those of female menopause. This is why the name has stuck, even though it is inappropriate, and has held up acceptance and treatment of the condition it describes. Not only were the symptoms clear cut, but the cause was shown to be insufficient testosterone for the body's needs, because the amount of testosterone which overflowed into the urine decreased with age and other hormones from the pituitary gland increased to try to stimulate its production.

Some of the most conclusive evidence comes from this period. A remarkably modern 'blind' trial was reported in the prestigious *Journal of the American Medical Association* in 1944.[8] There, testosterone injections were clearly shown to rapidly and dramatically relieve the symptoms of male menopause, while placebo injections of the carrier sesame oil did not.

An editorial in the same issue gave the official blessing:

The facts that are here cited serve to indicate with increasing probability that male climacteric is just as truly a syndrome based on endocrine disturbances as is menopause syndrome in women.[9]

In the same year as this medical recognition, an explanatory article in the *Reader's Digest Magazine* made it clear to the general public that the condition and its treatment were established facts. This was followed in 1945 by a powerful book by an American writer, Paul de Kruif, called *The Male Hormone: A new gleam of hope for prolonging man's prime of life*.[10] This detailed how theories relating to testosterone treatments rose and fell and rose again, and made a compelling case for its widespread use. Game, set and match to male menopause activists! What could possibly go wrong?

Well, fashions change. After a few years, more sensitive chemical tests were introduced which could measure the minute amounts of various hormones in the blood, including testosterone. It was then found that the total amount of testosterone in the blood of most men did not decrease much with age. It was therefore argued that while women at menopause showed a dramatic fall in blood estrogen levels which would account for their symptoms, men did not and therefore their symptoms must be imaginary.

Male menopause detractors also explained away its symptoms as the emotional upheavals of the 'male mid-life crisis.' The latter is an existential, emotional crisis, not a hormonal one, and the two need to be clearly distinguished. More on this later.

For the last 25 years, because of conflicting evidence surrounding male menopause theory, the majority of doctors have ignored or derided it.[11] With more up-to-date and detailed research information, and a reassessment of the mass of supporting facts which can be gathered from literature and recent clinical experience, however, I hope to reestablish the concept and the benefits of treatment once and for all. I am convinced it is an idea whose time has come.

Chapter one

The testosterone story

Hormones have a long, exciting and checkered history, and testosterone has the longest, most exciting and most checkered of all. This is part of the problem in getting male menopause accepted as a real condition, so let's look back to see where the maze of myths surrounding testosterone started.

Antiquity

Castration makes the eunuch

This observation, properly credited to primitive man, ushered in the dawn of hormone research.[1] To emulate one of Sir Winston Churchill's most famous sayings, 'Never in the field of human science was so much learned by so many by the removal of so little.'

As the American journalist Paul de Kruif put it in his historic book *The Male Hormone*, printed in 1945:

> From the beginning of human record, priests, saints, medicine men, farmers and sultans had been demonstrating how clear cut, sure and simple it was to take the vigor of animals and men away. How? By removing their testicles.[2]

(Incidentally, de Kruif is another example of the wayward march of medical science. He asks, 'Why didn't they reason that older men, losing their youth gradually, might also be suffering a slow, chemical castration taking place invisibly with the passage of time?' Then he goes on to document how the 'hormone hunters' aim to rescue 'broken men' by isolating and then synthesizing testosterone. However, his message had to wait 50 years to be heard.)

Castration carried out on young boys was always recognized as preventing the onset of puberty, with lack of body hair or beard, more feminine fat distribution and a high-pitched voice much valued in singing. This was thought to be worth the sacrifice by some Italian singers, the *castrati*, or at least their managers, as graphically shown in the film *Farinelli, Il Castrato*. Eunuchs were also known not to develop male pattern baldness and to be less muscular.

Depending on how long after puberty it was performed, castration also reduced the eunuch's sexual and other drives, as well as making him infertile, but did not invariably make him lose erectile power. The more potent eunuchs were used by Roman women, particularly when their husbands were away fighting for the Empire, for sex without procreation.

Eunuchs were also known to be less competitive and aggressive. For the 1,000 years from about AD 400, the Byzantine Empire was run increasingly by eunuchs, who were efficient, but predictably unadventurous and submissive. They also played an important part in the administration of the Imperial Court. They presumably knew their place and posed no threat to the Emperor or those vying for power.

Similarly, farmers of antiquity knew that castration could be used to fatten pigs, bullocks and cockerels to produce capons. The taming of wild animals for domestic purposes and tempering the fiery nature of both horses and dogs through castration made the psychological effects of this operation in other species equally apparent.

The great physician Hippocrates, said to have created medicine as both an art and science, lived during the golden age of Greek culture, born in 460 BC and living to over 90 years old. In the many classic writings noted by his pupils, he observed that gout does not appear before puberty, women do not develop it until after menopause and eunuchs not at all. Modern theory would suggest that the high levels of uric acid which cause this particularly painful condition of the joints come from the breakdown of the protein in the large muscle masses which testosterone produces in the postpubertal male.

Hippocrates also knew that mumps could be followed by the inflammation of the testes known as orchitis and then sterility. This can also contribute to an early onset of male menopause (*see pages 73–4*).

Judaic medicine meanwhile, derived from the Old Testament, held that health was the gift of God and disease his wrath. Ill health could therefore only be prevented by submission, atonement, prayer, moral reform or sacrifice. It was also recognized, however, that stress, disease, fatigue and starvation could reduce the amount of semen. These are all factors now known to lower testosterone levels, particularly in older men.

The Bible differentiated between those who because of diseased or undescended testes developed eunuchoid features (known in Egypt as 'those castrated by Ra,' the sun god, therefore 'sun-castrates') and those castrated by man ('man-castrates'). When castration was performed for religious reasons, the penis was often removed as well, a mutilation now only seen in some transsexuals.

The differentiation is described in Matthew 19:12, where Jesus is quoted as saying:

> For there are some eunuchs, which were so born from their mother's womb: and there are some eunuchs, which were made eunuchs of men: and there be eunuchs which have made themselves eunuchs for the kingdom of heaven's sake.

In the last category, he appears to be referring to priests who achieved celibacy without going to such extreme measures.

These causes of testicular insufficiency, or hypogonadism, are recognized today as either originating before birth or later in life following some damage to the testis or interference with the production or action of testosterone. The origins of male menopause mainly fall within the second category, but occasionally there are elements of early factors which have been overlooked, as when one or both testes fail to develop or descend fully. Then there may be sufficient hormone to take the boy through an apparently normal puberty and even make him fertile, but in his thirties or forties the other factors which contribute to menopause cause the limited supply of testosterone to become insufficient.

In India, from ancient times, those who renounce sexual activity because they believe it dissipates their spiritual energy have been known as *bramacharya*. In the Hindu tradition, this is one of the requirements of becoming a monk or Swami. A vegetarian diet may help them to make this difficult sacrifice and keep from straying from the spiritual path by decreasing the amount of cholesterol available for testosterone production.

This effect was confirmed in 1984 when a Swedish study showed that switching from a high to a low fat diet, particularly one high in polyunsaturates, lowered blood testosterone levels by 10 percent.[3] This makes sense in evolutionary terms, as the killer instinct of the hunter would be enhanced by the higher level of testosterone produced by having a higher fat, higher cholesterol diet than the more placid herbivorous prey.

When the beadle of the orphanage in the Dickens story Oliver Twist got into a fight during his apprenticeship to an undertaker, the head of the orphanage rebuked his employer with the words, *'You never should have given the boy meat. Meat heats the blood.'*

Perhaps, too, the old man who for many years used to wander up and down Oxford Street in London with sandwich boards denouncing the 'passion proteins' in meat and declaring that they led to war, may have stumbled upon an important truth.

Also, phytoestrogens, the estrogens present in many plants, can antagonize the effects of testosterone and give a more female type of fat distribution. The plants richest in these phytoestrogens are soy, particularly tofu and miso, citrus fruits, wheat, licorice, alfalfa, fennel and celery. This may be why some vegetarian yogis have enlarged breasts, a condition known as 'gynecomastia', and large abdomens. Pliny recorded 2,000 years ago that *'Hempseed and chondrion make men impotent.'* Also, heavy beer drinkers can have enlarged breasts and a 'beer belly' as well as the erection problems desribed as 'brewer's droop,' caused by the phytoestrogens in hops, along with the calories from the alcohol and its damaging effect on the testes and liver.

The most influential physician of Roman times was Galen (AD 130–200), who is considered the greatest medical man of antiquity after Hippocrates. He wrote more than 100 books, which dominated medical thinking for more than 1,500 years, well into the Renaissance period and beyond. However, he could also be thought of as the founding father of medical dogmatism because his system was so authoritative and rigid that it almost completely stifled fresh ideas throughout that time.

In spite of this, Galen could be considered the forerunner of sex hormone theory and research. He describes how the 'maleness' of men could cease with castration and the 'femaleness' of women with disease or aging of the ovaries. He noted that these sexual characteristics were generalized throughout the body in all the species he studied, and were not purely genital, being seen for example in the lion's mane, the cock's comb and the boar's tusk. These remote and widespread effects are the characteristic features of hormonal action.

Also, in his book *Peri Spermatos* ('On the Seed'), Galen raised a key question about the menopausal reduction of vitality: '*What is, therefore, the cause, that castrates slow down in their whole vital capacity?*' He remarks that castrated animals lose not only the power to procreate, but also the desire to do so, and that eunuchs showed the characteristic changes in normal male fat and hair distribution. In modern medical parlance, they show all the signs of testosterone deficiency.

The medicinal properties of semen

Linked to observations on castration was the idea, fairly common throughout antiquity, that semen was beneficial to men's health.

About 4,000 years ago the *Pen Tsao*, the Chinese 'Great Herbal,' recommended the use of the semen of young men for treating sexual weakness in the elderly, a remedy doubtless popular with the wives of the impotent potentates.

In India, the Hindu Ayurvedic system of medicine which developed from 1400 BC onward suggested the consumption of testicular tissue to treat impotence and obesity. It was also known at that time that hot baths could reduce fertility, which is still news over 3,000 years later.

Nearly 2,000 years ago, the Greek physician Pliny recommended eating animal testicles to improve sexual function. This remedy is still popular in many countries, especially Spain, where cooked bulls' testes are served as the delicacy known as *cojones*. Not coincidentally, this is also the Spanish word for courage. Unfortunately, any benefits obtained from eating such dishes are likely to be more morale boosting than hormone boosting, because although most of the body's supply of testosterone is made in the testes, it is rapidly exported to the rest of the body in the bloodstream, and there is little concentrated on site at any one time.

For example, when chemists first extracted the hormone from bulls' testes in the early 1930s, it took several tons to produce a few hundred milligrams, presently one day's dosage for a patient. This makes using this dietary source on a regular basis a daunting task! To make things worse, testosterone taken by mouth, unless it is in a special, easily absorbed and stable form, is broken down in the liver and never gets circulated in the body. This makes Pliny's treatment, although it must have sounded like a theoretically good idea at the time, practically useless – except for the doubtless strong placebo effect.

Later, the Roman physician Aretaeus, who gave the first detailed description of sugar diabetes, wrote:

> For it is the semen, when possessed of vitality, which makes us to be men, hot, well braced in limbs, well-voiced, spirited, strong to think and act.

He added, *'for when the semen is not possessed of its vitality, persons become shrivelled,'* which is a good description of the wrinkled skin and wasted muscles of the testosterone deficient male.

The renaissance

It was only with the wave of radical new thinking that swept through Europe at the end of the fifteenth century that medicine broke free of the bondage imposed on it by Galen's dogma.

This rebirth in both the arts and sciences was precipitated by two events. One was the fall of Constantinople in 1453, which ended the Byzantine Empire and caused many scholars to move to Italy. As a result there was a revival of Greek medical thought and the ideas and observations of Hippocrates.

The other was the information revolution started by the printing of the Gutenberg Bible in 1454, which soon spread to the production of medical texts. Let's hope that the new information revolution produced by the computer and the Internet, which is starting to give us access to medical databases all over the world, will produce even greater advances in freedom of thought on all medical subjects, including andropause.

One of my heroes from the Renaissance period is Paracelsus (1493–1541), or, to give him his full title, Aureolus Theophrastus

Bombastus von Hohenheim. He was the most important medical thinker of the sixteenth century. As his name suggests, he was a swashbuckling Swiss physician and chemist, who not only had the audacity to challenge Galen's ideas, but publicly burned his books. He revived Hippocratic thought and ideals in medicine and introduced many new ones of his own, especially in relation to thyroid disease. He died unloved and unrecognized by the medical establishment of his day, but left a legacy of original thought which led to fresh medical thinking and experimentation on hormonal factors in health and disease. His approach influenced, among others, Charles Darwin, who appealed to scientists to abandon intellectual 'idolatry.'

Paracelsus introduced a new vision of disease as a distinct explicable entity which could and should be treated. This was in opposition to the Galenic view that most conditions were untreatable and should be borne with fatalistic resignation. For example, Paracelsus successfully introduced mercurials for the treatment of syphilis, the most feared disease of the sixteenth century, which was viewed in the same light as AIDS today. Perhaps we need to invoke the spirit of Paracelsus to encourage a wider discussion of male menopause.

How did the intelligent public view aging in the male at that time? With his usual intuitive clinical accuracy, Shakespeare described the seven ages of man in his play *As You Like It*. We can now recognize how each age is influenced by the effects of testosterone:

At first the infant,
Mewling and puking in the nurse's arms.

In the infant there is no real difference between the testosterone levels in boys and girls, though intrauterine differences have left their physical and emotional imprints.

And then the whining schoolboy, with his satchel,
And shining morning face, creeping like snail
Unwillingly to school.

The surge of testosterone at puberty generates the rebellious male nature and increases skin oil or sebum, which makes the skin shiny and later, causes acne. The sexual characteristics of the adult male appear at this stage.

> And then the lover,
> Sighing like furnace, with a woful ballad
> Made to his mistress' eyebrow.

With the libido going full blast due to the peaking levels of testosterone, and rampant priapic power available, mating and nest-building activities normally tend to predominate now.

> Then a soldier,
> Full of strange oaths, and bearded like the pard,
> Jealous in honour, sudden and quick in quarrel,
> Seeking the bubble reputation
> Even in the cannon's mouth.

Plenty of testosterone still, making him belligerent and driving him through what is often a period of questing and hasty decisions, the 'mid-life crisis.'

> And then the justice,
> In fair round belly with good capon lin'd,
> With eyes severe, and beard of formal cut,
> Full of wise saws and modern instances;

With testosterone activity declining, the scene is set for male menopause to appear, characterized by weight gain and muscle deterioration seen first in the Elizabethan couch potato's expanding waistline.

> The sixth age shifts
> Into the lean and slipper'd pantaloon,
> With spectacles on nose and pouch on side,
> His youthful hose well sav'd a world too wide

For his shrunk shank; and his big manly voice,

Turning again towards childish treble, pipes

And whistles in his sound.

Now the decreasing free testosterone levels and lack of physical activity fail to maintain muscle mass, particularly in the legs, so that the calves and thighs shrink. Lack of testosterone also results in thinning of the vocal chords, which return to their prepubertal state, giving a higher pitch.

In the last scene of all, that ends this strange, eventful history,

Is second childishness, and mere oblivion,

Sans teeth, sans eyes, sans taste, sans everything.

Sadly, the old saying that what you don't use you lose comes true at this stage of life. There is considerable evidence to suggest, however, that testosterone treatment can slow the rate of physical and mental deterioration in this final stage, and help men to maintain both the will and ability to continue active life until they drop. You now have the choice!

The Eighteenth and Nineteenth Centuries

The dominant figure in experimental medicine in the eighteenth century was the English surgeon John Hunter (1728–93). Among his amazing range of original studies were the experiments supporting his view that sexual characteristics 'depend on the effects that the ovaria and testicles have upon the constitution.' He obtained evidence for this statement in a variety of ways.

He carried out an interesting experiment on how the testes enlarged during the mating season in a variety of animals, by killing and preserving a series of London cock sparrows at monthly intervals from midwinter to spring. Hunter's students later reported on his demonstration that:

The one killed in December has testes not bigger than a small pin's head, the rest are gradually larger, the testes of the last, killed in April, are as large as the top of your little finger.[4]

We now know that this seasonal growth of the testes, with the accompanying surge in testosterone, occurs because the longer days trigger the pineal gland at the base of the brain to switch off production of its 'hibernation hormone,' melatonin. This in turn causes the pituitary gland to produce more of the hormones which rouse the dormant testes to spring fever pitch. It seems, however, that bright city lights are now suppressing this seasonal cycle and causing mating activity in cosmopolitan sparrows all year round. Although in humans there is a slight surge in conception rates around holiday periods such as Christmas, there is a larger rise in late spring and early summer, so we still retain this link between sunshine and sex.

What has not been sufficiently recognized is that Hunter carried out transplantation experiments which showed that if the spur of a hen were transplanted to a cock, it would grow to the size of a cock's spur. He went on to demonstrate that if the small spur of a young cock were transplanted to a hen, it failed to grow at all. Also, in 1771, he transplanted cocks' testicles into their abdomens and observed that they continued to grow there. He transplanted them into the same site in hens, too, with some evidence of a masculinizing effect.

However, Hunter failed to publish his results, illustrating the truth of that old medical dictum 'Publish or perish.' It was not until over 70 years later, in 1849, that Adolf Berthold, a German professor at the University of Göttingen, who knew of Hunter's work, repeated the experiment, showing that capons could grow into normal cocks following testicular transplants:

> They crowed quite considerably, often fought among themselves and with other young roosters, and showed a normal inclination to hens.[5]

In particular, the transplants prevented shrinkage of the comb, restoring this dramatic red crowning glory which signals the male's sexual maturity. It was clear proof that the testis produced a substance which traveled in the blood to maintain the sexual characteristics of the adult male animal.

This first well-documented, successful hormone replacement therapy inaugurated a century of attempts to use testicular extracts or implants to rejuvenate men. However, most of these attempts were either of doubtful effectiveness, mainly relying either on the placebo

effect of giving patients a novel form of treatment or on fraudulent confidence tricks based on the instinctive wish for a long and active life. It
is difficult to this day to decide whether doctors offering rejuvenation
treatments are pioneers or buccaneers who navigate 'this poorly chart-
ed sea of medical research.' Time and future research will tell.

One who must certainly be regarded as a pioneer was the eminent
neurologist and physiologist Charles Edouard Brown-Séquard
(1817–94). He had a distinguished career in France, where he was
the successor of the celebrated physiologist Claude Bernard at the
Sorbonne in Paris, and held positions in England and America, as well
as being the first to demonstrate that the adrenal glands were essential to life.

However, his colleagues became critical of his ideas when in 1869
he suggested that 'the feebleness of old men is in part due to the
diminution in functions of the testicles' and:

> If it were possible to inject, without danger, sperm into the veins of old men,
> one would be able to obtain with them some manifestations of rejuvenation at
> once with respect to intellectual work and the physical powers of the organism.[6]

They were even more sceptical when in 1889, still actively researching
his ideas at the age of 72, he announced at a learned gathering in Paris
that he had mentally and physically rejuvenated himself with subcutaneous injections of extracts of the testicles of dogs and guinea pigs.
Within three weeks, the *British Medical Journal* had published a report
on his lecture criticizing his ideas and the manner of their presentation. Under the heading 'The pentacle of rejuvenescence,' it pronounced sarcastically:

> The statements he made – which have unfortunately attracted a good deal of
> attention in the public press – recall the wild imaginings of medieval philoso-
> phers in search of an elixir vitae.[7]

Similar responses to reports on the benefits of treating male
menopause are still prevalent over 100 years later. Looking back,
Brown-Séquard's ghost might well comment, '*Plus ça change, plus c'est
la meme chose.*'

In England and the rest of Europe his results were said to be due to autosuggestion, or even hypnosis, which was very fashionable in France at the time. He tried to counteract this notion by not giving the patients any idea of the results he was expecting, although any treatment by such a distinguished and imposing professor must have had some placebo effect.

He also sent his extracts to sympathetic colleagues in England and America. Although some reported good results, the general medical reaction in Britain was hostile to what rapidly became known as one type of 'organotherapy,' or treatment with glandular extracts or transplants. However, some of the critics were given pause for thought by work going on at the same time on the more obvious, reproducible and clear-cut benefits of treating thyroid-deficient (myxoedematous) patients with thyroid extracts.

In America, by contrast, the reaction to Brown-Séquard's work was overenthusiastic and the testicular extract was widely inflicted by charlatans on a gullible public as 'the Elixir of Life' for every type of ailment from senility to tuberculosis. This and other organotherapies became even more fashionable because of the simultaneous introduction of 'serotherapies' – the use of sera and vaccines of animal origin for the prevention and treatment of infectious diseases.

The failure of such extracts led to Brown-Séquard dying a discredited man. Moralists were quick to criticize his therapy, and the ridicule that it brought to the whole field of research into the hormonal functions of the testis has lasted to the present day. He *made the blunder that put the male hormone in the scientific doghouse,'* as Paul de Kruif points out.[8]

In Victorian England, matters relating to sexual activity were considered 'not quite nice' and unsuitable topics for research anyway. Even learned and very influential physiologists such as Sir Edward Sharpey-Schafer (1850–1935), who wrote many papers and a book on 'endocrine organs,' had a Freudian block about reproductive hormones and in a lecture on 'internal secretions' given to the British Medical Association in London in 1895 denied that the testes had any endocrine actions. It is amazing that so great a pioneer in other areas of endocrinology could have so complete a blind spot in this one.

Another testicular experiment with an unfortunate long-term result was performed in 1896 by two Austrian doctors who claimed that testicular extracts of bulls' testicles could improve the strength of their hand muscles. They concluded: *'The training of athletes offers an opportunity for further research in this area.'* This report foreshadowed the damaging influence that steroid abuse by athletes would have on the medical and public image of testosterone treatment.

The Twentieth Century

Endocrinology

The twentieth century heralded the birth of the science of hormones, or endocrinology. The word 'hormone' was introduced in 1905 by a British physiologist, Professor Ernest Starling, in a lecture he was giving at the Royal College of Physicians in London. It was derived by two scholarly professors at Cambridge University from the Greek verb *hormao*, meaning 'to put into quick motion,' 'to excite' or 'to arouse.' Starling used it to describe the 'chemical messengers' that were released into the bloodstream by the body's ductless or endocrine glands (*endon*, 'internal' + *krino*, 'to secrete'), such as the testes, thyroid and adrenals, from the external (*exo*, 'outside') secretions of glands with ducts, the exocrine glands, such as those that produce saliva or tears. The new science lived up to its name by making rapid advances which excited both the public and medical imaginations.

Typically the history of any one hormone goes through four stages:

First, there is the observation that a gland or organ produces an internal secretion that has a general effect on the body.

Second, methods of detecting the internal secretion and measuring its effects are developed. This is usually done initially by biological assay, to see what action the preparation containing the hormone has on an animal or organ lacking it. Later, chemical methods of measurement can be found.

Third, the hormone is extracted from the gland or organ and isolated in a pure form.

Fourth, chemists define its structure and synthesize it.

Testosterone was the first hormone to be recognized and measured, but because of the complexity of its molecule, the process of isolating and synthesizing it was relatively slow.

At the turn of the century, though, organotherapy, the use of extracts from different glands, particularly the thyroid and adrenal, continued to be the subject of much speculation and experimentation. However, it soon became clear that testicular extracts were not sufficiently powerful to have the effects originally claimed. This was because the minute amount of testosterone produced in the testes is continuously being swept away into the bloodstream and is not stockpiled in the gland.

Remembering the work of Hunter and Berthold, doctors then attempted what would be a difficult feat even today: transplanting testicles from man to man. In 1912 and 1913 two apparently success-ful operations took place in America. The second of these was per-formed by a Dr Victor D. Lespinasse of Chicago, who reported the full restoration of libido and sexual function over a two-year period in a man previously without sexual desire and impotent from the loss of both testes.

The First World War then held up endocrine research and prevent-ed communication between doctors working in different European countries for many years. However, an interesting report emerged that the famous Danish surgeon Thorkild Rovsing had carried out an experiment that indicated testicular function might be important in relation to circulation, as Brown-Séquard had claimed. After a young soldier had been killed in battle, Rovsing transplanted his testicles into an old man with gangrene, which then, according to the case report, healed completely.

In 1918 the resident physician in San Quentin prison in California, Dr Leo L. Stanley, who had access to many fresh testicles 'donated' by executed prisoners, started transplanting them into other inmates of various ages.

Some of these regained their sexual potency, although how this was measured in the prison is unclear – and freedom is a great aphro-disiac. Two years later, because of 'the scarcity of human material,' even in that situation, Stanley moved on to transplanting the testes of rams, goats, deer and boars into his rapidly expanding patient population. These testes, perhaps suspiciously, seemed to be equally effective. Interestingly, as with Rovsing, gangrene was among the wide range of conditions, from senility to diabetes, which Stanley's treat-ment claimed to benefit.

In the early 1920s, a flamboyant Russian-French surgeon working in Algiers, named Serge Voronoff, made his fame and fortune by transplanting chimpanzee and baboon testicles into humans, and claimed they had powerful rejuvenating effects. This work naturally attracted great medical and public interest, and international deputations of doctors as well as patients from many countries made the pilgrimage to Algiers to investigate Voronoff's 'monkey gland' treatment.

If Voronoff was just fooling people, he did so with a lot of detailed evidence and seemingly convincing results for at least a decade. Even my first professor of physiology at the Middlesex Hospital in London, Samson Wright, described Voronoff's work in detail in his standard textbook of 1926:

In successful cases it is claimed that very striking results are obtained from this operation. Old people, with marked signs of senility, are claimed to be thus transformed into vigorous energetic individuals. Previously castrated persons may regain their secondary sex character – e.g. growth of beard and moustache may occur.[9]

He obviously took this work seriously:

While Voronoff's operation appears quite justifiable in young subjects in whom the testes have been damaged or destroyed by injury or disease, the treatment of senility by this method is more questionable. We have no proof whatever that senility is solely due to atrophic changes in the testis; it is almost certain that many other factors are concerned. Though the testicular graft may stimulate physical activity and sexual desire, it cannot restore the worn heart, arteries and essential organs to their normal state. There is a grave danger that excessive strain may be put on damaged structures, with disastrous results.[10]

These same lines of argument are still used today by doctors urging the fatalistic 'do nothing' option.

Pure testosterone

As the war clouds cleared in Europe after the First World War, a great pharmaceutical arms race developed with three drug companies competing to be the first to produce the active ingredient of the testicles in pure chemical form. It is an amazing example of synchronicity that after a search for the essence of manhood lasting over 4,000 years, the three different groups passed the finishing line within four months of each other.

First, on May 27, 1935, was Ernst Laqueur, a professor of pharmacology in Amsterdam, who led an excellent research team for the Organon drug company. He emerged triumphant from a veritable mountain of bulls' testicles with a few precious crystals, submitted a paper called 'On crystalline male hormone from testicles' and coined the name 'testosterone' for it.[11]

Second was a formidable, dynamic German chemist with a dueling scar on his left cheek, Professor Adolf Butenandt. He was working for the Schering Company in Berlin, which had managed to survive the First World War with its manufacturing capacity intact. In 1923, thanks to hyper-inflation it made a profit of 286 million billion marks, after tax, giving the shareholders a dividend of two billion percent. Some of this profit it invested in collecting 25,000 liters of policemen's urine, enough to fill an Olympic size swimming pool. From this, Butenandt, with bravery clearly above and beyond the call of duty, extracted 15 mg, a few crystals, of a relatively inactive urinary breakdown product of testosterone called androsterone.[12]

He then decided that this method of preparation was too much like hard work and thought up the much more commercial way by which testosterone is made to this day. He methodically worked out its structure and then produced it, as does the body, from cholesterol, its natural precursor. He sent his paper on this process and the structure of testosterone itself to the German Journal of Physiological Chemistry on August 24, 1935.[13]

Just one week later, a Swiss chemical journal received a paper from Leopold Ruzicka, a Yugoslavian chemist working for the Ciba company in Zurich, announcing a patent on the method of production of testosterone from cholesterol.[14] For this work, he and Butenandt received the Nobel Prize in 1939.

Within two years of these momentous discoveries, a variety of testosterone preparations were in clinical use. It was soon found that because it was an oily substance which didn't dissolve readily in water, it couldn't be absorbed by mouth in its pure form. So a slow release form that could be given by injection, testosterone propionate, was synthesized and soon became widely used. This proved very successful in patients whose testes were insufficiently active for a variety of reasons, including those showing signs of male menopause.[15] Like insulin injections for diabetics, which had been introduced 15 years earlier, it was dramatically effective in restoring the two big Vs in men's lives: Vitality and Virility. Now that you could 'get it in a bottle,' testicular transplants and extracts went out of the window.

Studies on patients throughout the late 1930s and the 1940s showed a wide range of benefits from testosterone in medical conditions ranging from heart and circulatory problems, including gangrene, to diabetes.

Although the injections lasted about three days, another longer lasting form of testosterone was also introduced. Compressed crystals were fused together to form pills and later small cylindrical pellets which under local anesthetic could be implanted under the skin of the buttock or abdomen. This was both effective and convenient as the implant continued to act for six months.[16] Sixty years later this is still one of the best methods of giving long-term testosterone treatment. There are few medical preparations, particularly in endocrinology, which have stood the test of time so well.[17]

A third type of preparation, also made in the early years of testosterone treatment, was a water-soluble form called methyl testosterone.[18] Unfortunately, although it was effective in relieving symptoms, this form proved very toxic, especially to the liver. Nevertheless, its widespread use for over 50 years, often as under-the-counter gold and silver covered pills that were claimed to have almost magical sexual powers, has done a great deal of harm to the safety image of testosterone. It is amazing that even today, when testosterone's dangers have long been recognized and it has largely been taken off the market throughout the rest of the world, it is still almost the only form of oral testosterone available in the USA, where several safe derivatives cannot be marketed.[19]

Unfortunately, in Britain, this toxic drug, known as Prowess, is still being manufactured and sold in capsules, also containing the supposed sexual stimulants yohimbine and pemoline. Such toxic products should be banned by international agreement.

Testosterone used to treat male menopause

From 1940 onward, mainly because of the obvious improvements brought about by testosterone, many doctors accepted that there was a group of symptoms commonly experienced by men in their fifties similar to female menopause or 'climacteric,' from the Greek word *klimacter*, meaning 'the rung of a ladder,' and therefore a critical period in a man's life when the vital force begins to decline.

An outstanding paper of this time, which used testosterone as definitive proof of the existence of male menopause, was published in the prestigious *Journal of the American Medical Association* in 1944. 'The male climacteric: its symptomatology, diagnosis and treatment' was written by two American doctors, Carl G. Heller and Gordon B. Myers.[20] It is well worth looking at this historic paper in detail, as the case has seldom if ever been better made.

The symptoms which the authors attributed to the male climacteric were exactly those of male menopause: loss of libido and potency, nervousness, depression, impaired memory, the inability to concentrate, fatigue, insomnia, hot flashes, and sweating.

They began by listing all the points raised by those who were skeptical of the existence of this condition and then used their clinical studies to answer them one by one. The majority of these points were based on the general view that no objective evidence had been put forth to prove menopause was an actual clinical entity, or to differentiate it from neurosis or impotence of purely emotional origin. Also, many men remained fertile to an advanced age and did not show the marked physical changes that menopausal women showed.

To study this, Heller and Myers developed a measure of testicular function based on the hormonal feedback mechanism which controls the production of testosterone in men and estrogen in women. When the amount of active testosterone or estrogen drops, the small pituitary gland at the base of the brain, which is in overall control, releases more of two hormones – gonadotrophins, so called because they stimulate these sex glands. When the activity of the sex hormones increases to the point where they are adequate for the body's needs, the gonadotrophins fall to a low level.

Nowadays gonadotrophins can be measured by sensitive chemical tests on the blood, but in the 1940s Heller and Myers had to extract urine samples from men taken after a 12-hour overnight period, inject the extract into immature female rats and measure the increase in the weight of their ovaries caused by these hormones. This simple biological test gave surprisingly clear-cut results. The urine of normal men, or those whose symptoms were due to anxiety or neurosis, showed virtually no gonadotrophin activity in the urine. Those whose symptoms were due to a true male climacteric syndrome showed high levels of urinary gonadotrophins, as demonstrated by the ovaries of the test rats doubling or trebling in size.

This carefully performed and detailed study gave unequivocal evidence that male menopause was a physical fact, not just a fiction created by the emotionally disturbed and neurotic. Also, when a therapeutic test was carried out on samples of both groups of men by giving injections of testosterone propionate, the neurotic group 'experienced little, if any, improvement in potency or in well-being.'

By contrast, in the male climacteric group they reported that:

Definite improvement in the symptomatology was noted by the end of the second week in all of the twenty cases treated. Complete abolition of all vasomotor, psychic, constitutional and urinary symptoms was accomplished by the end of the third week in 17 of the 20 cases treated. In the remaining three cases vasomotor and urinary symptoms were abolished but the psychic and constitutional symptoms persisted in spite of continuation of treatment for several months and doubling the dosage for brief periods. It was concluded that these three persons were suffering from involutional melancholia [depression of old age).

The same study also answered a frequent criticism of testosterone treatment which still comes up today, that it will restore libido but not help problems with erections, thus leaving the patient more frustrated than before. Heller and Myers' experience coincides with my own:

Sexual potency was restored to normal with these doses in all but two cases, in one of which involutional melancholia was present.

They go on to remark that with increased dosage, *'Sexual vigor in both previously refractory cases exceeded that of normal men.'*

They further gave evidence that this is a real response to testosterone treatment and not just a placebo effect:

In 14 cases therapy was subsequently withheld for from four to fifteen weeks and in all instances the symptoms returned and sexual potency was again lost. On resumption of the therapy with testosterone propionate, relief of symptoms was again afforded and sexual potency returned. Thus the specificity of therapy was established.

To investigate further the possibility that the improvement may have been due to suggestion, placebo injections were administered. Ampoules containing 1cc of sesame oil, packaged similarly to the original testosterone propionate, were substituted without the patients' knowledge in several cases. No improvement was noted in any case.

As well as recommending pellet implants for long-term treatment, Heller and Myers made two final important points in this historic paper. These were that *'the male climacteric is not confined to middle and old age but may occur as early as the third decade'* and their conclusion:

Whereas in the female menopause is an invariable and physiologic accompaniment of the aging process, in the male the climacteric is an infrequent and pathologic accompaniment of the aging process.

We will see later why male menopause may have become more common half a century on and yet is still not being properly diagnosed or treated.

Dr Tiberius Reiter

Starting in 1950, Dr Tiberius Reiter, a German physician who set up a private practice in London's exclusive Harley Street, used testosterone pellet implants to treat men in their forties, fifties, sixties and seventies suffering what he called 'IDUT syndrome.'[21,22] These initials indicated the main features of the condition: impotence, depression, urinary disturbances and thyroid overactivity. Included in the latter were irritability, headaches and attacks of rapid heartbeats, particularly at night, which just about completes the classic picture of male menopause. Reiter attributed all these symptoms to testosterone deficiency.

For over 20 years he treated more than 350 patients, with very good clinical results. These he wrote up in considerable detail in a series of eloquent articles, carefully documenting the improvements in each symptom on his own rating scale. As well as being the first to actually measure lowered testosterone levels in his patients before treatment, he emphasized the safety of testosterone and suggested that far from being dangerous, it showed evidence of benefiting the heart and prostate gland.[23] He also wrote a monograph for Organon, the company who made the implants, describing his method of implanting testosterone pellets into the buttocks.[24] These are the method and materials I continue to use in some cases for long-term testosterone treatment, and they provide a powerful, safe and effective way of giving the hormone.

From the recollection of his medical colleagues, several patients and his widow, Nancy Reiter, an interesting picture emerges of this remarkable man. He was a dynamic, charismatic individual who delighted in the improvements he saw in his patients. He believed in a broad approach to treatment and would sometimes take his patients to his favorite fish restaurant to teach them at a pleasant practical level the benefits for virility of eating oysters, with their high zinc content. As Nancy put it, he was regarded with *'plenty of skepticism from the medical world – but the patients kept coming!'*

Reiter was well received in America, where he published three articles in the *Journal of the American Geriatrics Society* between 1963 and 1965. In 1965 he also lectured at their 22nd Annual Meeting in New York City, receiving considerable interest and approval.

However, in Britain he remained an unrecognized prophet. Despairing of getting his message across, he devised a cunning plan. He went to a meeting on endocrinology at the prestigious Royal Society of Medicine, the heart of the medical establishment, in Wimpole Street, London, and at the question time at the end, stood up to deliver a long fiery diatribe about the virtues of testosterone treatment. When the chairman finally managed to shut him up – which took some doing – he went to the front entrance of the imposing building and met a group of journalists he had previously summoned. He then gave them full details of his learned address to the Royal Society, which were duly printed, together with his picture, in the newspapers that evening.

Perhaps not surprisingly, such direct action did not endear Reiter to academic doctors, but he died in 1972 much loved by his patients – truly another hero of the hormonal revolution.

Dr Jens Møller

Another of the great pioneers of testosterone treatment was the Danish doctor Jens Møller. With all the fire and tenacity of his Viking ancestors, he fought a 30-year war against the medical establishment in Denmark and throughout Europe for its use. I had the privilege of working with him during the last 10 years of that war and it was he who in 1977 first interested me in testosterone.

At the time I had been working as Senior Lecturer in Chemical Pathology at St Mary's Hospital Medical School in London. Although my office and research laboratory were located within the department of Professor Vivian James, one of the world's leading researchers on steroid biochemistry, which includes the study of testosterone, estrogens, cortisol and other related hormones, I was more excited by the stress hormones such as adrenaline and noradrenaline which appeared more directly related to stress, tension and heart disease, my main area of research.

However I was very interested in exercise as a means of balancing the effects of stress and protecting the heart from them. As part of this program of research, I was taking part in a study set up by the Medical Research Council at the City Gymnasium in London. The founder and owner of this gymnasium was an ex-Olympic weight-lifting coach called Alistair Murray. With tremendous energy and enthusiasm, he originated the use of vigorous but not violent exercise in the form of circuit training for the prevention and treatment of heart disease in

London businessmen. We had just written a book together for the British Sports Council called *F40: Fitness on Forty Minutes a Week*,[25] based on his ideas and reporting this research.

One day while I was at the gym Alistair called me into his office to meet a tall Dane. Though friendly, this doctor had a military bearing and the charm of a diplomat which he could switch on or off at will. When it was off he could be what he described as *'very direct.'* He was then in his seventies, although he had the brisk manner and energy of a man 20 years younger. As I learned later, he had had a varied career demonstrating the power of any mention of testosterone treatment to excite extreme passions – in the minds of medical men.

Born in North Jutland in 1904, Møller left home at 16 and became a successful entrepreneur, working in Paris, London and Berlin. Even with money to burn, however, he found his business career meaningless, and at the end of the Second World War enrolled at the university medical school in Copenhagen, getting his entry qualifications in three months rather than the usual year. He qualified five years later, at the age of 50, and began his medical career, which was to be as unusual and turbulent as his previous one in business.

After a variety of work in hospitals and the pharmaceutical industry, he decided he wanted to be a neurosurgeon and worked in Sweden for a time. As neurosurgical jobs were few and far between, he took a locum job with a private physician working in Copenhagen, a decision which was to alter the course of the rest of his career.

Doctor Tvedegaard, whose name I shall abbreviate to Dr T., was already a controversial figure in Danish medicine because of his use of testosterone to treat severe arterial disease, particularly in the legs. He had studied its use by German doctors and seen amazing results even in the most severe cases of gangrene.

The typical history given by his patients was of painful cramps in their calves when walking, especially uphill on cold days, a condition known as 'intermittent claudication.' As the blood supply became worse, the pain gradually became more continuous, even at rest and in bed at night, so that the patient would have to hang his leg out of bed to ease the intense discomfort. Eventually the limb would stay cold and blue most of the time, and even an otherwise trivial injury to the foot would turn into an infection leading to gangrene of one or more toes. According to conventional practice at the time, these would then have to be amputated and the surgeons would start on what often turned out to be a series of amputations, nibbling their way up one or both legs to above the knee.

Testosterone injections, often in considerably higher doses than generally prescribed, seemed to halt, or in some cases even reverse the otherwise inexorable process at almost any stage. Walking would be prolonged because the cramps in the calves would come on later and later, and even disappear, leaving a very happy wanderer. Night cramps would also go, which greatly improved the quality of sleep. Cold, blue, painful feet and legs would become pink and comfortable as the circulation mysteriously improved. Even gangrene would heal without surgical intervention, much to the relief and delight of the patients and their relatives. Although this did not necessarily prolong their lives, it did give them a much better quality of life and could prevent them becoming crippled by their circulatory problems. Many were the patients who went happier to their graves with two whole legs rather than one or none as the result of this testosterone treatment.

At the time this was very strange and inexplicable. However, even more curious was that instead of other doctors becoming interested in this treatment, investigating it further in an open-minded spirit of scientific inquiry and perhaps even trying it on some of their more severe cases, who after all had nothing to lose except their legs, the reverse occurred. Because testosterone treatment did not fit the medical orthodoxy of the time, was not recognized in the groves of academia and was a dirty foreign product originating in still deeply detested Germany of all places, Danish doctors closed ranks and minds against it. It seemed that the rigid, doctrinal, Galenic attitude had once again triumphed over the investigative, clinical, Hippocratic one.

Although burning at the stake (other than intellectually) had gone out of fashion, doctors still managed to find ways of dealing with troublesome medical heretics. Suppressing their ideas by turning down their papers for medical meetings and publications was a good start. If theories are not published or discussed, they can't be any good, can they? Not surprisingly, Dr T.'s three papers for Danish medical journals were rejected.

Dr T. was often outspoken and critical of his colleagues' attitude and made many enemies among them. So when an opportunity for discrediting him presented itself, it was eagerly seized.

In Denmark at that time the law relating to medicines said that conditions could only be treated with the drugs officially recognized as being effective in those disorders. Because of prevailing medical opinion, not only in Denmark but in most other countries as well, testosterone was not on the list of drugs to be used for circulatory problems. Even if an army of 1,000 people whose limbs had been saved marched up and down outside the Danish Parliament for a week, the law was the law, and medical opinion could not be moved to change it for sweet reason's sake.

Also, patients could have some of the costs of certain 'vital medicines' refunded, provided the condition for which they were given was on the authorized list and the prescriptions were written on the appropriate red forms. Dr T felt deeply that testosterone was a literally lifesaving 'vital medicine' and, because it came mainly from the testes, he found a category of 'genital insufficiency' which he thought qualified its use in the cases he saw and daily wrote his prescriptions on red forms.

Unfortunately, in August 1957 this came to the notice of Danish Health Service officials, who 'saw red' and reacted in a surprisingly dramatic fashion. Rather than take the case up through the usual medical disciplinary channels, they sent the state police around the same day to officially charge Dr T. and Dr Møller with betraying the Government for money, because testosterone was not a 'vital medicine.'

This rapidly escalated into a very public *cause célèbre* with many court hearings. Questions were asked in the Danish Parliament. Dr T.'s health soon deteriorated under the strain, so Dr Møller, who was made of sterner stuff, was left holding the testosterone baby.

Undeterred by rulings against them in the courts, he mobilized public opinion in their favor. He did a detailed study of the literature and went to Germany to discuss the use of testosterone with the leading endocrinologists of the day, who were very supportive of his ideas. He then organized a public meeting of over 1,500 patients and relatives to raise funds for the fight. He lined up doctors from the health authority in the front row, deluged them with this new scientific evidence and then said, '*Contradict me if you can.*' They couldn't, and left the hall in a state of confusion and acute embarrassment.

The fight then got very dirty. The police tried to seize all the patients' case notes and deprive the defendants of their evidence. Dr Møller took the case notes home and piled them in the fireplace, telling his wife to set fire to them if the police showed up while he was out. The prosecution even made up stories from patients about how they had been treated. Fortunately, many grateful and influential patients kept up the legal battle. Literally their lives and limbs depended on it.

Finally, after two years, a Minister of Justice who was on the State Medical Ethics Committee and had a close relative who had been greatly helped by Dr Møller's treatment got the court's decision reversed and the case called off. Not only that, but the Director of the Danish Health Authority, who had been one of Dr Møller's fiercest opponents, saw the effects of the treatment on his family and friends, and changed his mind to the extent that he became Director of LBK, an organization which was set up to promote the use of testosterone.

The facts in this amazing case are documented in a book called *The Tvedegaard – Møller Trial: A fight against injustice* written a year later by another Danish doctor who had supported their cause.[26]

Although the medical establishment in Denmark generally remained hostile to the 'Dr Tvedegaard treatment,' which they used to tell their students was '*hormonal humbug*,' Dr Møller's practice flourished. He used to see 50 or more patients a day and sometimes they had to line up in the street outside his clinic in the fashionable Store Kongensgade (Great King Street).

As is traditional with native prophets, Dr Møller began to receive much more recognition from abroad than in his own country. Many distinguished doctors from America, Britain and all over Europe visited his clinic, but Danish medics seldom came to call except when they wanted research funds from Møller's rapidly growing charitable foundations.

Not unnaturally, these experiences left Dr Møller feeling somewhat paranoid, and it became his mission for the rest of his life to hammer home the message of the effectiveness and safety of testosterone. To this end he established the European Organization for the Control of Circulatory Diseases, or EOCCD, at a meeting of the European Parliament in Strasbourg in 1976 and enlisted many prominent politicians as well as doctors in his fight against what he called '*the international enemy*' of circulatory problems.

From 1977 onward I made many visits to his clinic in Copenhagen and saw for myself the dramatic benefits of testosterone treatment to the circulation, especially in the legs. I came to realize some of the good effects of testosterone and helped Dr Møller to edit the books he was writing,[27,28,29]

I also went with him as he raced around Europe in his capacity as President of the EOCCD, holding meetings in London, Luxembourg, Strasbourg, Bonn, Berlin and Munich. We visited many eminent authorities throughout Europe and Dr Møller achieved a great deal of scientific support for his ideas. It was difficult to keep up with him even when he entered his eighties and it soon became apparent that he certainly took his own medicine, which was as effective for him as it was for his patients.

When he finally died in 1989, active until the end, he left thriving national and international organizations which are continuing his work under the direction of his able successor, Dr Michael Hansen. This seems a fitting guarantee that Dr Jens Møller's heroic work in the service of testosterone will continue to bear fruit.

My own experiences in trying to prove the existence of male menopause have closely mirrored those of many of the characters featured in this story, particularly Paul de Kruif, Dr Tiberius Reiter and Dr Jens Møller (see chapters 10 and 11). Attempts to debate the condition and its treatment with other doctors, especially those in related specialties such as endocrinology and urology, have met with what could best be described as blatantly illogical denial. This has been laced with emotion and rhetoric far exceeding the spirit of detached scientific debate. Interestingly, the family doctors with whom I have had the opportunity of discussing the subject, both individually and in teaching seminars round the world, have been much more inquiring and open-minded in their response than the specialists.

It seems that history is likely to repeat itself, as it often does, and that testosterone replacement therapy for men will arrive by the same route as estrogen replacement therapy for women. It was the enthusiasm of the women themselves which gathered converts to the cause, not the recommendations of doctors. Only after several years of intense opposition, including predictions of doom and disaster from the majority of gynecologists, did doctors generally become supportive of those seeking treatment. The situation has now changed to the point where the majority is in favor and a few doctors have become downright evangelical – while still remaining generally hostile to the idea of similar treatment for men!

A poll in a major British national newspaper in 1996 established that 97 percent of its readers believed that male menopause was a fact and should be treated. However, in the same month at a meeting of urological specialists at St Bartholomew's Hospital in London, only one third agreed the condition existed and even fewer considered that treatment might be safe or effective.

To enable you to decide whether this is a fictitious or real condition which should be treated, let's now look at the experiences of some of the thousand or so patients I have seen over the last 25 years with symptoms they put down to male menopause and the benefits they received from testosterone treatment.

Chapter two

Male menopause or andropause

What's in a name? In the case of male menopause, a lot. It is probably one of the main reasons why the condition has failed to achieve the recognition it deserves.

For the sake of clarity and brevity, and to ease acceptance by both the general public and the medical establishment (who already recognize the name, if not the disorder), I will now mainly use the term 'andropause' when referring to this condition in men and 'menopause' when referring to the equivalent condition in women.

After all, the term 'menopause' was introduced by French doctors in the 1870s, combining two Greek words – *menses* ('periods') and *pausis* ('stop') – to indicate the time in a woman's life when monthly periods stop, just as the word 'menarche,' combining *menses* ('periods') and *arkhe* ('start'), means their beginning. When applied to men, the word is therefore both inaccurate and, because of its effeminate overtones, somewhat derogatory. One of the aims of this book is to change that image and make the whole subject easier for men to talk and think about.

'Andropause' combines two Greek words – *andro* ('male') and *pausis* ('stop') – and means 'when masculinity ceases,' which is a much more accurate description of the condition. It is doubly appropriate because the root of the problem is an inadequate supply of androgens, the hormones which provide manliness (*andro*, 'male,' *gen* 'give'), and which can be used as an effective remedy for the problem.

Women are used to visiting their gynecologist – *gynaeco* ('female'), *logist* (scientist) – to sort out their problems. I suggest that men should be equally willing to consult their 'andrologists.' These practitioners are beginning to have an expanded role beyond male fertility to include the particular health concerns of men and are now in a good position to advise on testosterone replacement therapy to treat andropause.[1]

Let's start with a brief sketch of the condition, how it begins and how we can recognize when it happens to us or those around us. Its often insidious onset can be at any time from the age of 30 onward, although typically it is in the fifties. One reason it's often missed is that it usually begins more gradually than menopause does, although it is more severe in its long-term consequences. It is a crisis of vitality just as much as virility, even though its most obvious sign is loss both of interest in sex and of erectile power. Surprisingly this change is often overlooked or ignored, either because the man is so pressured by the rest of his life that he assumes it is an inevitable part of growing older or because his sexual partner has lost interest as well.

Besides lack of sex drive, there is often loss of drive in professional or business life, so that the leader becomes the led, the lion becomes the lamb.

There is usually also fatigue, lethargy, exhaustion and depression, accompanied by a sense of hopelessness and helplessness. All too often men change their jobs or their women – anything to ease the malaise they feel – usually with little relief. Sometimes things are made much worse because of the additional stress these changes bring.

Physically, there is commonly stiffness and pain in the muscles and joints, or symptoms of gout and a rapidly deteriorating level of fitness. There may also be signs of accelerated aging of the heart and circulation.

Typical of andropause case history is that of John:

I'm just 50 now and I've been very successful in my family's retail business. Because of the recession it is harder to make a living than it was, and work is stressful and not much fun.

My health has always been pretty good, except for one attack of prostatitis associated with a urinary infection five years ago. This 'non-specific urethritis,' as they called it, had me up peeing five to ten times a night until it was treated with a four-month long course of antibiotics, but it seemed to clear up completely.

After that, however, although I loved my wife and we had a good life and four delightful children, my libido just faded away to nothing compared to the healthy sexual appetite I had for our previous 25 years of happy married life. I've never been one to have affairs, but then I wasn't even interested in 'window-shopping.' I just felt cocooned and detached from even the prettiest girls, as though I wasn't in the same world as them!

My erections weren't great either, and I had more and more failures in that department, especially when I was tired or had had a few drinks. Morning erections were few and far between, and my wife isn't really turned on at that time. Sex between us was down from two to three times a week to once a month, especially as I didn't like to go into battle if I wasn't sure my guns would fire. In some ways I didn't miss sex that much, although my wife did, just as you don't miss food if your appetite has gone.

Worse still, I completely lost my drive and ambition over those five years. When I got up in the morning, I felt 'energyless' and completely lethargic, and instead of looking forward to the day, I just wondered what time I could get back to bed. I was really envious of older people with more energy than me. I wasn't giving much time to my wife or the children, which made me feel guilty about them, especially as I was usually as grouchy as a bear with a sore head, and that's not like me.

There were physical changes in me, too. My feet and ankles, knees and back were very stiff in the mornings, which made me feel old and decrepit, and even less like getting out of bed. Often the bed was sopping wet in the mornings because I sweated a lot more than I used to and sometimes this was so bad that my wife had to change the sheets. I found that I flushed easily when the room was warm, but that my feet and hands were cold most of the time. What with that, the night sweats and the lack of sex, my wife was threatening me with single beds!

I don't go to my doctor often, but a year or so ago I went to see him, feeling thoroughly depressed and convinced that something must be wrong with me. He's a good fellow and heard me out sympathetically. But when I said that I thought that my symptoms were just like my wife had had before she went on hormone replacement therapy and wasn't there something similar he could give me, he nearly threw me out of the office! I was told to forget it and given a choice of antidepressants or marriage guidance counseling, or both, but I didn't feel either of these were right for me.

Just as I was getting desperate, my wife saw an article in a magazine about male menopause being a real condition that could be positively identified and

safely treated with testosterone. She said the case described was an exact pic-
ture of me. I went through the appropriate tests and safety checks, and started
on testosterone capsules by mouth. Within two weeks the symptoms had
improved and within a month they had gone. My marriage, my family life and
my business have all benefited. I feel like I did 10 years ago. My wife and I
would like to know why did I have to have all those wasted unhappy years when
my hormone deficiency could have been detected and fixed so easily. It seems a
reasonable question to ask.

I spend a lot of time going over men's case histories the first time
they come to my office and they mainly tend to be variations on the
same theme. No one symptom is essential, but the picture is consistent enough usually to be able to make the diagnosis even before
examining the patient or doing the detailed blood tests.

Based on the histories of over 2,000 men who have been to see me
over the past 15 years and a detailed analysis of the symptoms shown
by the first 1,000 of these, I have built up an 'identikit picture' of the
andropausal male. See if it fits anyone you know.

The main complaints can be mental, such as fatigue, depression,
irritability and reduced libido, or physical, such as aging, aches and
pains, sweating and flushing, and failing sexual performance. You can
see how close the comparison is with menopause in women.

Let's consider these symptoms one by one in more detail so that
you can recognize andropause when you see it coming. Above all,
remember it is usually treatable and, as it says on the front cover of
Douglas Adams' *Hitchhiker's Guide to the Galaxy*, 'Don't Panic!'

Fatigue

Fatigue is the main expression of the loss of overall vitality which char-
acterizes andropause. In my first series of 1,000 men it was present in
nearly 80 percent of cases. It's as though the man's get up and go has
got up and gone. This is hardly surprising if you look on andropause
as a hormone deficient state. Remember the word 'hormone' comes
from the Greek for 'setting in motion.'

The patients very graphically describe this drop in energy levels and
its return after treatment, as in Bruce's case:

Fifty was a turning point for me. Until then I had been pretty active as an
advertising executive, but at that time I just seemed to grind to a halt. I felt

tired at work, couldn't concentrate, lost my competitive edge and found my job more and more difficult. Partly this was because I was getting more and more short tempered, and I started drinking fairly heavily in the evenings.

At home, I wasn't exactly a bundle of fun either, falling asleep on the sofa every evening. Although everyone told me I needed a good vacation, I was so tired and negative and the interest and energy needed to organize one just didn't seem to be there. My libido had dropped to the point where even a 'Saturday night special' was usually too much trouble, especially as my erections let me down increasingly often. This was all very depressing, especially when a close friend about my age suddenly died of a heart attack.

After having had these symptoms for four years, my marriage was falling apart and I seemed likely to lose my job. Then I read an article in a magazine and felt the author was writing about me, he described my symptoms so exactly. It all seemed so unfair as there wasn't anything in my medical history that I felt was relevant and my family doctor had told me that I had nothing but a touch of depression. However the tests clearly showed a low 'free testosterone' and I started right away on capsules to boost levels of the hormone.

The results were dramatic. Within a month I felt as though the treatment had lifted a veil over my life, and I felt generally more vibrant and more virile. After three months my performance at work was back up to speed again and in managerial jargon I was more 'proactive.' Also, both at home and at work I was rated 'Mr Nice Guy.' My sex life has improved and my wife is delighted with the results of treatment. Things are going well across the board and, feeling more positive about myself and life in general, I have gotten on top of the alcohol problem, just having a moderate amount of wine at home over the weekend and none during the week.

Conventional female wisdom has it that it is not the man in your life that matters, as much as the life in your man. What is the life in your man? It is the testosterone drive. This is probably the most important force underlying both mental and physical energy. The ability to reproduce by sexual activity is the essential biological function of all animals, the biological imperative, subordinate only to the needs of staying alive long enough to do it and insure survival of the offspring.

Many and varied are the ritual tests of manhood. Full-scale battles and individual combat for love, honor and leadership are as old as mankind itself. In Germany ritual dueling with swords, inflicting facial scarring, was fashionable before the Second World War. In Spain, young men still show their bravery and impress the girls by running in front of the bulls in the streets of Pamplona. Triumphant racing drivers world-wide enjoy the heady symbolism of spraying champagne over adoring crowds. In America, depending on the amount of money available (which is a form of financial testosterone), you arm wrestle, play 'chicken' by riding motorcycles at other young men down the middle of the road or drive your Ferrari Testarossa as fast and as dangerously as you can. Either way hormones have the last word, often literally.

Testosterone, then, is what drives men on for a large part of their lives and, along with intelligence, is often the deciding factor in their social and sexual history. It can be thought of as the 'success hormone.' When a man is winning life's battles it is high and when he's losing it falls. When it gives out on him, and his drive in both bedroom and board room fades, he goes onto 'emergency power' and cuts down on all nonessential activity. At home, sex goes out of the window and both social and domestic activities dwindle and die away. All this sets up enormous tensions and resentments within the entire family. The worsening cycle of failures and recrimination tends to disturb sleep and is made worse if a less than sympathetic wife keeps the husband awake by reciting his escalating list of errors of omission and commission.

After a bad night, the man goes to work feeling 'lower than a snake's belly,' drained of energy and enthusiasm. If he tries to regain some by drinking endless cups of coffee, these may just make him more nervous and irritable and raise his anxiety levels even higher. His attention span and ability to concentrate also deteriorate, as does his memory. Not only is he unable to think up new ideas or put them into action, but his ability to sell himself and his projects also slumps.

Unfortunately, customers and competitors alike have an unerring ability to spot when a man is down and out of testosterone, even when he is trying his hardest to put on a brave face. Body language can give clues – does the man slouch in with an apologetic, round-shouldered, crouching look or stride in, standing tall, with his shoulders back and arms outstretched, looking and feeling great? Is his voice high-pitched, wavering and anxious or low-pitched and steady? Pheromones, those airborne hormones derived from the sex hormones and given off by the skin all over the body, but particularly the genitals and armpits, may also give the game away. They can either send out the sweet smell of success or the sour scent of failure.

One famous captain of industry in Britain, Sir John Harvey-Jones, when prodded in the midriff with a pocket tape recorder by writer, Gail Sheehy, researching the subject of male menopause, urbanely replied that he felt sure there was such a condition. He said he had often seen previously dynamic, hard-driving, successful managers *'go off the boil,'* as he put it, sometimes with disastrous consequences for them or their organizations.

Sir John Harvey-Jones felt that he had been through one such 'fallow period' in his own career around the age of 50, but had fortunately come through it spontaneously. He went on to suggest that the careers of men who ran into such problems could often be saved, with great benefits to the companies for which they worked, if ways could be found to help them through such difficult times.

All too often, however, during a recession, a company will fire the andropausal man whose performance is dropping without inquiring, or him admitting, the reason for this drop. To make the situation worse, this frequently happens at the same time as the man is 'fired' from the marriage bed for also underachieving at home.

Depression

Variously described by patients as 'negative' or 'low' mood, depression is one of the most common features of andropause and, in my first series of patients, was present in 60 percent of cases.

Although only rated as mild to moderate on one of the standard psychiatric rating scales used in the study, it was one of the most difficult of the symptoms for the men and their families to live with. After all, together with life and liberty, the pursuit of happiness is written into the American constitution, and most of the patients didn't feel up to pursuing anything, especially happiness.

Colin's story is typical of their experiences:

Eight years ago the bottom dropped out of the stock market and my life at the same time. First my investments went, then my beautiful country home and finally my job as a promoter. There were plenty of reasons to be depressed, but I felt sure I had something more than just a natural reaction to all these problems. My brain felt full of what I can only describe as toxic sludge. I couldn't focus on anything and was very irritable, as well as being tired and weepy.

Going along with my doctor's view that it was just plain depression, I went to see a psychiatrist who tried me on every antidepressant under the sun, including Prozac, but without success. As a hopeless case, I was threatened with electro-convulsive therapy, but protested and was let off with psychotherapy, which got me into tears and then anger in a big way.

Just when I'd given up hope, there was an article in a magazine which talked about hormonally-based depression in 'male menopause.' A light went on in my head when I read how the combination of the vasectomy 20 years ago, when I was just 30, and the large amounts of alcohol taken to blunt the pain of my financial ruin might have made my depression very much longer and more severe by affecting my testosterone levels.

My doctor fortunately, was open-minded enough to encourage me to take the tests and they showed twice the usual level of a binding protein in the blood which, as he explained it, was 'tying up' my testosterone so very little of it was active.

On the hormone treatment, the depression gradually lifted over three or four months. Six months later, my energy and drive have doubled, and I'm employable again now. I still occasionally suffer bouts of depression, but they are much shallower and quicker to recede. I'm back on an even keel again much more rapidly now and looking forward to life being plain sailing again after the terrible storm which nearly sank me.

Depression can be very destructive. It can make a man even less optimistic at work and less likely to suggest, start or carry through new projects. At home, it can not only cast a black cloud over the whole house, but also narrow the social horizons. This can continue to the point where the andropausal man never goes out to visit family or friends, who soon get the message that he doesn't want to see them. He is usually to be found slumped in front of the television in a torpid heap. All of this causes the social support inside and outside the family to break down.

Nervousness, anxiety about everything and everybody, and lack of self-confidence often go hand in hand with the depression, as was recognized in studies of the 'male climacteric' 60 years ago. It can also be accompanied by sleep problems, both in getting off to sleep because of intrusive thoughts and worries and in the early waking characteristic of depression. Unfortunately sleeping pills may just make the tiredness worse during the day and contribute to erectile problems at night.

Although after years of depression a man may reach the point where he feels tired of life, fortunately he often doesn't even have enough energy for suicide!

Sometimes it is difficult to tell which came first, the depression or the other symptoms, since if you are severely depressed, tiredness and loss of libido and potency can result. However, only in a very small proportion of my cases was the depression severe enough to account for the other symptoms.

Most of these cases had already been treated with antidepressants without improvement – some had even become worse. This is because antidepressants can make feelings of tiredness worse and the majority seem to interfere with erections (although fortunately, there are exceptions, *see pages 133–4*). Personally, I don't usually use any anti-depressants until testosterone treatment has been tried on its own for three to six months, unless the depression is exceptionally severe and life, job or marriage threatening. This is because my original ratings showed, and my consistent experience is, that TRT on its own gently but firmly lifts the depression, often completely, at the same time as it relieves the other andropausal symptoms.

Irritability

One of the most distressing symptoms of andropause is irritability, both for the men suffering from it and their families. This behavior can be entirely unusual for the person concerned or represent an even shorter fuse in somebody with an already low flash point.

Trivial issues will irritate the man, as much, if not more than important ones. At work, the firm suddenly starts to recruit nothing but idiots, then trains them to work against him and there are no dirty tricks they won't try. At home the whole family deliberately tries to annoy him and succeeds brilliantly! They do all the wrong things at all the wrong times in all the wrong ways. Without having to try, he gets into endless arguments with them and ends up infuriated, his patience, like the rest of him, utterly exhausted. He may well be aware that he is being unreasonable and be ashamed of it, but still be unable to do anything about it.

Bernard describes this well:

I suppose it all began when I contracted mumps at the age of 26. This was one of the most serious illnesses I had experienced. My testicles became swollen, so much so I could hardly walk. I had to wear a support just to go to the bathroom. Every footstep was agony. I also lost a couple of days. I was delirious and remember very little. Three to four weeks later I was almost back to normal, although one testicle was smaller than the other. Nothing seemed to have been adversely affected and, while not ravenous, my sexual appetite seemed normal.

Several years later, around the age of 40, I seemed to be experiencing a number of things. First and foremost I was irritable, irrationally moody and intolerant of other people. The supermarket checkout was constructed just to annoy me. The salesperson was an idiot and out to obstruct me. The other car driver was a moron and should never have been given a license. They were all trying to cut me off, get in my way and generally make life difficult for me. I invented both 'shopping cart rage' and 'road rage!'

On top of this, my sexual appetite was zero and I often failed to get erections. My wife by this time was convinced I was having an affair. It all added up – no sex and an attitude to boot! Finally my wife gave me the ultimatum: see a doctor or we split. A week later I had an interview and a blood test which confirmed a hormone deficiency and that treatment would be appropriate. I was prescribed a course of testosterone capsules which I started immediately.

Ten days later I was a changed man. I felt a tremendous burden had been taken from me. I felt energetic, I became more assertive and I had regained my sexual appetite. My job became easier, I made decisions more easily and I had the energy and determination to see things through. I felt more optimistic and no longer had this feeling of frailty or vulnerability. My erection was much stronger and didn't fail me at the crucial moment. My attitude changed; I returned to being the laid-back, happy and contented person I had been. No more anger, no more moods. I could now enjoy life instead of feeling angry as it passed me by.

Ten years later I'm still on the treatment. My job hasn't changed very much but I can handle it much more easily and confidently. I am more successful at doing what is needed. I've gained a lot of self-confidence and I'm not at all susceptible to bouts of depression. My family life is very much happier and the relationship between myself and my stepson has moved much further forward. My wife and I have regained our loving relationship and our sex life is much more satisfactory to both of us.

Time after time stories like this completely go against the idea of testosterone being the hormone responsible for male aggression and violent behavior. Usually what is often described all too literally as 'impotent rage' is associated with *low* levels of testosterone activity. When they are restored to normal by treatment, the man feels more confident and assertive, and this doesn't seem to overshoot into aggression.

At home, however, the family may have become used to having a human doormat around, and the marked change may not always be welcome as the new man puts his foot down.

Reduced libido

The word 'libido' means sex drive or sexual appetite and is the same word in Latin, where it was taken to mean 'desire' or 'lust.' One thing that men and women have in common is that their level of libido at any one time is governed by the higher centers in the brain and conditioned by life experience, social factors and hormones, principally testosterone.

This is surprising, since men normally have about 20 times the testosterone level of women, but although men may set the ball rolling more often, most couples usually end up agreeing on the level of sexual activity between them. Extreme exceptions to this such as when a man is a multiple rapist or a misogynist, or a woman a nymphomaniac or totally frigid throughout her life, are nearly always due to psychological causes rather than hormonal ones.

However, because the baseline level is so much lower in women, relatively small variations of testosterone may cause big swings in libido. For example, at the middle of the menstrual cycle, when the woman is ovulating and at her most fertile, there is a surge in her testosterone level to put her in the mood for sex.[2] Women who are more assertive and take up more traditionally masculine roles in society such as lawyers[3,4] or business bosses have been found to have higher testosterone levels and frequently are sexually more active.[5] Complaints of sexual harassment of male employees by their female bosses, unheard of a few years ago, are becoming relatively commonplace.

Though the factors affecting libido are complex (for more information, see the series of books *The Disorders of Sexual Desire* by the American sexologist, Dr Helen Singer Caplan), many women with low libido, particularly around the time of menopause, can be helped by carefully administered low dosage testosterone. If the dose is excessive, not only may masculinizing effects such as increased facial hair and enlargement of the clitoris occur, but the libido may become excessive. The Australian feminist Germaine Greer described on a television program how she was put in an embarrassing situation when a doctor gave her too much of a long-acting testosterone compound and she suddenly found out 'what a rapist felt like.' This had the unfortunate effect of being one of the factors which turned her against the use of HRT in women, as argued in her book *The Change*.[6]

A group of American women who call themselves 'The Third Sex' deliberately take high doses of testosterone. Despite having to shave hair all over their body frequently and getting shrinkage of their breasts, they figure that the overall buzz they get from it, and the almost insatiable sexual appetite that goes with clitoral enlargement, makes it worth the chemical sex change.

With andropause, one of the commonest complaints, present in 80 percent of cases, is a reduction in libido. This usually comes on gradually over a period of months or years, as the level of active testosterone wanes. If the onset is sudden, or related to a particular event such as illness, the arrival of the first child in the family or the discovery that the partner is having an affair, a physical or emotional cause is suggested rather than a hormonal change. However in extreme cases one can lead to the other.

The fall in libido affects every aspect of a man's sex life, reducing the frequency of sexual thoughts, fantasies and even dreams. The number of times he feels in the mood for sex goes down and the partner may be convinced, usually entirely wrongly, that he has gone off them, is having an affair, or both. This can often cause problems in the relationship, which further saps the libido, because it can be difficult to be sexually turned on by an angry partner.

In nearly half the cases, the partner's libido then joins the downward spiraling of desire. The 'chemistry of charisma' seems to dictate that as a man's desire decreases, so does his desirability. So then neither party thinks it worthwhile to seek help.

In the most extreme cases, even the most beautiful, attractive or available of sexual partners fails to raise the slightest sexual interest. What Noël Coward called that 'sly biological urge,' is no longer working and his song of 'Let's do it' becomes 'I won't dance – don't ask me.'

Reduced potency

Reduced potency, in terms of obtaining or maintaining an erection, is one of the most distressing symptoms of andropause and occurs in about 80 percent of cases. The word 'potent' comes from the same Latin word meaning 'to have power, strength, ability or authority' or 'to be able to achieve the sexual penetration of a woman and to father children.' So a potentate is a ruler or a monarch who leads any group or endeavor, and has the power and position to rule over others. In many Eastern countries it is traditionally accepted that a ruler can have many wives or mistresses to demonstrate his position of dominance. When it becomes known that his sexual vigor is falling, his fall from power soon follows.

So, with potency seemingly the very essence of masculinity, its lack usually makes the sufferer feel much less of a man in all areas of his life. He is often more ashamed of this than any other symptom. And just using the modern medical parlance of 'erectile dysfunction' doesn't help a lot when the blunt fact of the matter is that in all senses of the term you can't get it up or keep it up, and you feel down about it!

The onset of erection problems is usually gradual and often starts insidiously with fewer early morning spontaneous erections, or 'morning glories' as some people call them. As the comedian Robin Williams, who himself looks like a regular high testosterone 'High-T Guy,' quipped in one of his shows, the penis is usually up and on parade five minutes before you are in the mornings. Indeed, it can be compared to a stand-up comedian: if he has a few bad shows, and worse still gets booed by the audience, he gets nervous and doesn't want to stand up and do his act. This is appropriately called 'performance anxiety.'

Although usually brief, these spontaneous morning erections are an important sign that the erection mechanism is working properly and has been primed by the testosterone surge which normally occurs around waking time. Their loss in andropausal men is probably due to the overall decrease in free testosterone which I have found to be the key diagnostic feature and by the reduction in the daily variation of testosterone levels with increasing age observed by me and reported by other researchers.[7] This view is supported by the fact that early morning erections are one of the earliest signs that potency has been restored by testosterone, and often happen within a week or two of starting treatment.

Another way in which erection problems begin is with occasional failures after a few drinks or when tired or stressed. Then they become more regular events – or nonevents, depending on which way you look at it. The progress of the problem is frequently erratic and depends to some extent on the attitude of the partner. If the partner is encouraging and supportive, and willing to help by trying massage, oral sex or different positions, the problem may not progress or may even be temporary. With an uptight, dismissive and hypercritical attitude, however, performance anxiety soon sets in. After several such put downs, a man is likely to shut down altogether. Nothing is more destructive to the male ego than criticism of either his ability to drive a car or to make love.

It is made even worse of course if news of his shortcomings is leaked to friends. This is why men are reluctant to own up to having this problem, even when talking to their best friend or their doctor. They try to laugh off the idea of there being any such condition as male menopause because it is too threatening to their self-image as potent males. Yet nowadays there are a whole range of methods, including testosterone treatment in particular, which, especially when combined with Viagra (see Chapter Eight), can relieve this particularly distressing symptom of andropause.

Further problems occur because the erection starts more slowly, is more difficult to maintain and often lasts a shorter time. Sexual activity may often be rushed and be less satisfying for women, who are often slower to become aroused and to reach orgasm, especially when they are post-menopausal. Anxiety makes the situation worse and can lead to premature ejaculation. A quarter more of my patients complained of this need to hurry to completion while they still had an erection. Alternatively, because of the decreased sensitivity of the penis which seems to occur in low testosterone states, there may be delayed ejaculation, as was experienced by another quarter of my patients.

Another factor contributing to this problem is the lack of tone and development in the pubococcygeal (PC) muscles around the urethra and base of the bladder. These contract, as do the corresponding PC muscles around a woman's vagina, during orgasm. Like other muscles in the body, with testosterone inactivity and lack of use, their contractions get weaker and, as the patients put it, the earth no longer moves for them or their partners.

Reduced penile size, particularly when erect, sometimes accompanies severe testosterone deficiency and can also become a problem for both partners. Although it is often said that size doesn't matter, most males are acutely aware of the usual size of their penis, both flaccid and erect, and get very upset if their vital statistics are reduced.

Research has finally caught up with experience when considering women's views on penile size. Although in the 1960s, Masters and Johnson, the American sexologists, tried to make out that a woman's pleasure and orgasm were solely due to the little bundle of erectile tissue and nerves called the clitoris, the man who can only deliver stimulation there is likely to be operating in an erroneous rather than erogenous zone. '*Vaginal sensitivity is an anatomical reality*,' says John Perry, a clinical sexologist. While there may not always be a distinct, raised G spot, the higher part of the front wall of the vagina, especially close to the urinary passage, the urethra, is richly endowed with nerves that play a major part in helping a woman reach orgasm. Part of the secret of sexual satisfaction therefore is to have this area stimulated by the tip of the penis. This can be achieved by having the right size penis in the right size vagina or by varying the position to improve penetration.

As well as reducing the firmness of pressure on both the clitoris and G spot, testosterone inactivity can shrink the penis to the point where partners who have been physically compatible in this area throughout a long and mutually enjoyable sexual relationship gradually become incompatible, to the distress of both.

Although to some extent it can be regarded as natural for the frequency and firmness of erections to reduce gradually with age, it is rapid acceleration of the process over a few months or years which should be thought of as abnormal and certainly worth investigation by the andrologist.

The causes of erectile problems are many and varied, and by the time the patient comes for treatment, several overlapping factors are usually present at the same time. There may be narrowing of the arteries by which blood is pumped in to expand the penis. There may be too much blood leaking out of it through aging veins, like a leaky bicycle tire. There may be poor nerve control, as with diabetes or as a side effect of tranquilizers, antidepressants or the drugs used to treat high blood pressure. Also, there are certainly likely to be relationship problems, as well as the dreaded performance anxiety.

A very broad approach is therefore needed to treat what may seem like a simple mechanical fault and important as I believe such treatment is, it is not just enough to throw testosterone at the problem and hope it will go away and stay away. To do the job properly the whole man has to be screened and a range of treatments appropriate for that patient needs to be administered.

Premature aging

To a great extent andropause can be thought of as a form of premature but reversible hormonal aging. I believe that TRT offers great hope in preventing, as well as treating, many of the conditions associated with advancing years in the male.

Heart

Generally you're as young as your heart and brain, which largely depends on how good the circulation is to these two vital organs.

When HRT for women was first cautiously introduced over 30 years ago, doctors feared it might contribute to diseases of the blood vessels and if a menopausal woman had even a family history of heart trouble, let alone cardiac disease herself, they said HRT was not for her. Much to their surprise, actual experience has shown the opposite to be true. Women on HRT suffered half the number of heart attacks of women who weren't. So, with some reluctance, doctors have begun to change their tack and say the treatment is positively indicated in women prone to heart disease.

The situation is the same with testosterone. Over the last 50 years, most doctors, including cardiologists, have taken the view that testosterone must be bad for the heart for two totally fallacious reasons. First, under the age of 50, men have five times as many heart attacks as women in most Western countries, although the women catch up soon after that age unless they are on HRT. According to this line of reasoning, therefore, testosterone is bad for the circulation and estrogen is good. Secondly, as already explained, because of the uniquely bad effects of the most commonly used preparation taken by mouth, methyl testosterone, and its abuse by athletes taking the wrong drugs in the wrong doses for the wrong reasons, anabolic steroids have had a very bad medical and consumer press. I used to share these views too until I met Dr Jens Møller. He led me to see testosterone as a very important and beneficial hormone for preventing and treating heart and circulatory problems. It was truly a case of seeing the light on the road to Copenhagen!

Several studies both from Britain and America have more recently shown lower levels of testosterone, and sometimes higher levels of estrogen, in patients who later developed heart disease than in normal control subjects the same age.[8,9] Other studies have shown the benefits of testosterone and related compounds in treating a range of circulatory problems, from ulcers on the feet to strokes in the brain (see Chapter 11).[10]

Circulation

Fortunately, the circulation problems experienced by the typical andropausal patient are relatively mild, and limited to cold feet and hands, especially in winter. What confuses the issue still further, however, is that the smaller blood vessels also become less stable in their reactions to heat, cold, alcohol, and other stimuli. Men with this condition can experience attacks of feeling a redness and warmth in the face, which may spread to the skin of their neck and face in warm surroundings or after drinking alcohol.

Although less common than in menopausal women, these 'hot flashes' can be very marked and acutely embarrassing.[11] Imagine how a senior executive feels when he stands up to make his key presentation at a sales meeting and starts by going beet red, as though he is deeply ashamed of his pitch. This is made even worse by the andropausal tendency to sweat profusely, so that the man ends up looking both hot and bothered.

Although less than a quarter of the men I originally studied had hot flashes, about half complained of increased sweating, especially at night. This could sometimes be so severe that not only the pyjamas but also the sheets were drenched with sweat. Some of the men felt they might have caught these symptoms from their menopausal partners!

Muscles and bones

Another common symptom of andropause is a general feeling of deteriorating physical condition. This is partly due to the decrease in muscle bulk and strength which accompanies the reduced level of testosterone activity. Also there are often diffuse aches, pains and stiffness both in the back and in many joints in the body, particularly the hands, ankles and knees, causing the 'Frankenstein syndrome,' as the first few creaking steps are taken in the morning. These are remarkably similar to the joint symptoms experienced by many menopausal women. They closely mimic arthritis, but fortunately usually show dramatic improvements with hormone treatment.

Osteoporosis, the thinning and weakening of the bones which causes older people to lose height from shrinkage and even collapse of the vertebrae, known as the dowager's hump in women, is also a source of much pain, unhappiness and disability in men. It is generally not as common or severe as in women and tends to come on later in life, from 70 onward. It mainly affects the spine, where it causes back pain and stiffness, especially in the neck, and the hips, where it contributes to osteoarthritic degeneration and sometimes fractures. It has been linked with low testosterone levels in general[12] and reduced free testosterone in particular.[13]

These symptoms are made worse, and the osteoporotic process probably accelerated, by the reduced muscle size and strength which accompany the reduced activity of testosterone which occurs in andropause.[14] Testosterone and exercise are the two main factors controling muscle mass and strength in the male. Together with calcium and protein supply, they also have an important effect in maintaining bone mass and strength.

This is why many andropausal men complain of a general deterioration in their level of physical fitness. It is particularly noticeable if they have previously been used to high levels of athletic performance. Those who like to work out in a gym notice that the amount of work they can perform in a session decreases, together with the number of push-ups or sit-ups. They also find their strength, in terms of the weights they can lift, goes right down. This, together with the decrease in muscle bulk that causes the pectoral muscles, biceps and thigh and buttock muscles to lose their hard-earned splendor, as well as the overall lack of drive and motivation, may even make the man give up exercise just when he most needs it.

Hair

Hair is another area of male vanity affected by andropause. The condition of the hair and scalp, and possibly its color, is affected by testosterone. In the andropausal male the hair is often dull, dry and lifeless, with a tendency to dandruff. The patient may say he is going grey very quickly. Baldness in men, however, is almost entirely hereditary and if a man's hair is going to go, it will happen whatever his testosterone level, unless he has been castrated before puberty.

Although the amount of hair on the chest is also hereditary, it is affected by lifelong testosterone levels. Sometimes, if it is very much reduced and the man only has to shave once or twice a week, it can indicate a life-long insufficiency of the hormone. But just because a man has typical male pattern baldness and plenty of hair on his chest does not mean, as is frequently assumed and quoted even by doctors who should know better, that his testosterone activity is normal.

On testosterone treatment it's interesting that some men notice a return of color to their hair. A few have even been accused by friends and relations of using hair dye. Many notice the improved condition of the hair and scalp. Also, more hair may appear on the chest, back and pubic region, which improves the man's image of his masculinity.

Fortunately, testosterone treatment does not accelerate the rate of balding and may even slightly slow it down.

Skin

Like the hair, the skin is sensitive to the action of testosterone. One of the ways in which the hormone is excreted from the body is as the sebum which normally oils the skin, and makes us more water resistant and drip-dry. This is why when teenagers get a pubescent surge of testosterone, they often suffer acne from blocked pores choked with surplus sebum. This also is sometimes seen in athletes overdosing on anabolic steroids.

In the andropausal male there is insufficient sebum and so the skin, particularly on the face and hands, is noticeably dry in nearly half the cases. There may also be thinning of the skin as collagen production is decreased, which makes it look thinner and more wrinkled. Again, this process is reversed by TRT and the person often appears to have more supple skin with less dryness, glossier, less brittle hair and even no more dandruff.

This wide range of mental and physical symptoms of andropause often feels like the onset of old age and cause great alarm. The man feels he is definitely over the hill and going fast down the other side. It doesn't help if his doctor dismisses him with 'It's your age.'

It's my goal in writing this book to make the point that although age may be one of the causes of andropause, a lot of other factors are involved, and in most cases a great deal can effectively and safely be done about it!

The first thing is to make the diagnosis and the second is to treat the condition. In my experience, the patient and his partner are often as good, if not better, than the doctor in deciding when andropause has arrived. Many of my patients were referred to me by their wives, who had accurately assessed their symptoms, related them to their own experience of menopause and in some desperation asked if there was any equivalent to the hormone treatment which had given them so much benefit.

Let's recap at this stage with a brief list of the symptoms of andropause and compare them with the menopausal symptoms in women:

Symptoms of female menopause

MENTAL	PHYSICAL
Reduced libido	Sexual enjoyment decreased
Fatigue	Aging
Depression	Aches and pains
Irritabilty	Sweating and hot flashes

Symptoms of male menopause (Andropause)

MENTAL	PHYSICAL
Reduced libido	Sexual performance decreased
Fatigue	Aging
Depression	Aches and pains
Irritability	Sweating and flashes

Andropause is often, as you will see from the comparison above, just as obvious as female menopause and essentially the symptoms are the same, but to serve as a more detailed guide I have designed the following 'Andropause Checklist,' which is a shortened version of the one I use in my clinic, and on the AndroScreen.com website.

This will enable you to determine with a fair degree of probability whether you or a friend or a partner are andropausal, although only assessment by a doctor experienced in this field and a full hormonal profile will confirm or exclude the diagnosis.

Andropause Check List (ACL)

	None	Slight	Medium	Severe	Extreme
1. Fatigue, tiredness or loss of energy	—	—	—	—	—
2. Depression, low or negative mood	—	—	—	—	—
3. Irritability, anger or bad temper	—	—	—	—	—
4. Anxiety or nervousness	—	—	—	—	—
5. Loss of memory or concentration	—	—	—	—	—
6. Relationship problem with partner	—	—	—	—	—
7. Loss of sex drive or libido	—	—	—	—	—

		30s	40s	50s	60s	70s+
8.	Erection or potency problems	——	——	——	——	——
9.	Dry skin on face or hands	——	——	——	——	——
10.	Excessive sweating, day or night	——	——	——	——	——
11.	Backache, joint pains or stiffness	——	——	——	——	——
12.	Heavy drinking, past or present	——	——	——	——	——
13.	Loss of fitness	——	——	——	——	——
14.	Feeling overstressed	——	——	——	——	——
		30s	**40s**	**50s**	**60s**	**70s+**
15.	The age you feel	——	——	——	——	——
TOTAL CHECKS		——	——	——	——	——
Multiply checks in each column by:		0	1	2	3	4
TOTAL SCORES		——	——	——	——	——

If there has been adult mumps, orchitis or other testicular problems, a prostate operation or inflammation, persistent urinary infection or vasectomy, each adds four points to the total scores.

TOTAL ANDROPAUSE SCORE ——

ANDROPAUSE RATING: 0–9 UNLIKELY, 10–19 POSSIBLE, 20–29 LIKELY, 30–39 VERY LIKELY, 40+ SEVERE

Chapter three

Not the mid-life crisis

Although male mid-life crisis may precede or even overlap male menopause or andropause, both are essentially separate and distinct conditions. In popular writing, however, they are still usually lumped together, which causes much confusion and prevents proper consideration and understanding of either.

The word 'crisis,' coming from the Greek *krisis*, meaning 'decision,' suggests a time of change, transition and opportunity. It also has the meaning of a turning point or crossroads. It's like the half time in a football game, when the manager tells the team to change their game plan if they want to win.

Many people decide that they either have no need or desire to make dramatic changes at mid-life and so the crisis may go unnoticed. Others face agonizing decisions that push them close to the edge emotionally, physically or financially.

What's your mental picture of the male mid-life crisis? Like male menopause, it's often seen as a joke. It's when middle-aged men temporarily lose their minds, leaving their wives, their jobs, everything that they had worked for up to that point in their lives, and running off in search of new lives and loves.

There is even a party game simply called MID-LIFE CRISIS made by Games Works, Inc. which is very amusing and informative about the subject. The objective of this board game for '2-6 adult players in their prime' is 'to get through your middle years with more money, less stress and fewer divorce points than your opponents or to declare a MID-LIFE CRISIS, in which case you must go broke, get divorced and crack up before anyone else reached the end of the game.' If you are in the danger zone of age 35-45, or have survived this and want to look back and laugh, I recommend it to you.

In 1973, an article by Dr M. W. Lear neatly summarized the dilemma of the archetypal middle-aged male:

> The hormone production levels are dropping, the head is balding, the sexual vigor is diminishing, the stress is unending, the children are leaving, the parents are dying, the job horizons are narrowing, the friends are having their first heart attack; the past floats by in a fog of hopes not realized, opportunities not grasped, women not bedded, potentials not fulfilled, and the future is a confrontation with one's own mortality.[1]

This last point, about looking at the hourglass of life and seeing that so much of the limited sand of this lifetime has run through, has been taken up by several novelists, including Martin Amis in his book *The Information*.[2]

This examines the competitive interaction – it can hardly be called 'friendship' – between two middle-aged writers. Like Amis, they are just turning 40, and are filled with extreme misgivings and 'comprehensive anxiety.' Both are living lies, one successfully, the other not. One has an unexpected best-selling novel on his hands and is riding high on his success, enjoying his money, public adoration and a titled wife, and looking and feeling good for his age. The other is floundering, feeling and looking washed-out mentally, physically, socially and financially. He has been working on a novel called 'Untitled' for several years, which is till unpublished. 'Stacked against him in the future, he knew, were yet further novels, successively entitled "Unfinished," "Unwritten," "Unattempted" and, eventually, "Unconceived."'

What makes it worse is that despite the totally disastrous and humiliating response when he eventually manages to get his book published, this man still believes in his ability as an author, whereas he is sure the other 'can't write for anything.'

This exploration of life's unfairness unfortunately fails to offer solutions to what in Amis's words is a 'terrible state, that of consciousness.'

Causes of mid-life crisis

Let's take a serious look at the causes of what I believe is a genuine and sometimes profound emotional crisis in a man's life, and how they differ from male menopause or andropause.

Many patients with the classic picture of andropause give an equally characteristic story of a series of events precipitating a mid-life crisis some five to ten years earlier. It is important to differentiate between the two conditions because the confusion between the two means that they are often lumped together and laughed off as a temporary emotional crisis without any physical cause. They are then considered to be just an excuse for men to behave badly toward the women in their lives, and to avoid their social or family responsibilities.

While male menopause is mainly a hormonal condition due to insufficient testosterone activity, as described earlier, it can also have profound emotional effects. The male mid-life crisis is essentially emotional in origin but if severe enough or long enough may have physical consequences, especially if alcohol or drugs are used to blunt the pain of the crisis.

Typically, the age group most prone to the male mid-life crisis is between 35 and 45. This may occasionally overlap andropause, which usually starts around age 50, although it can sometimes be earlier or later.

Many, if not most, mid-life crises go unnoticed and are passed off as the effects of a change of job, a change of house or a change of spouse. Only occasionally does the crisis turn into a drama, as can be seen daily in the lives and biographies of public figures, showbusiness personalities and politicians.[3,4,5,6,7]

In 2001 there seems to be two main celebrities contending for the male 'Mid-Life Crisis of the Year' award. In both cases, their lives seem to imitate their art. Hugh Grant, a classic contender, is described as 'single, famous and forty,' having broken off his long-term relationship with Liz Hurley. At the same time he is undergoing an image transplant, having moved from 'Mr Nice Guy' in 'Four Weddings and a Funeral' and 'Notting Hill,' via the changeable 'Mickey Blue Eyes,' to the cynical Daniel Cleaver character in 'Bridget Jones's Diary.'

Tom Cruises's seemingly inexplicable divorce from Nicole Kidman at the age of 38, undertaken with his 'Eyes Wide Shut,' must also put him in the running for the award. In Stanley Kubrick's last film, Cruise and his wife played a couple exploring the bounds of sexual fantasy within their marriage. For Cruise, this seemed to mark a turning point in his life from action hero to man on a quest, a wanderer searching for the real meaning of life beyond fame and fortune.

Both he and Hugh Grant typify the 'sex symbol hits identity and relationship crisis' model. In no way should it be confused with the low-testosterone, low-sexuality, low-drive, male menopause sufferer as happens in so many media muddles whenever the symptoms are mentioned. For a film representing male mid-life crisis, think of Kevin Spacey in 'American Beauty'; for male menopause think of Michael Douglas in 'Falling Down.'

What makes a man prone to a full-scale mid-life crisis? Well, anything that destabilizes him from childhood onward. This can include having a sensitive or artistic nature, distant or unloving parents, the losing of one parent, particularly the father, at an early age, losing or separating from a loved one or role model and repeated failure or, paradoxically, repeated success in his career.[8] As Oscar Wilde said, 'In this life there are only two tragedies. One is not getting what one wants, and the other is getting it.'

There may be an existential crisis in which the man may feel he is stuck in a career which either under-extends or overextends him so that he is faced with burnout. He may also be in a dead-end job or in a marriage that has become stale, having to choose between staying in that relationship or facing the trauma of divorce, particularly the pain of separation from his children, and the stress of starting over again financially. All this may lead to the 4D syndrome: depression, drink, drugs and divorce and set the scene for andropause which follows.

Differences between mid-life crisis and andropause

Let's run through a checklist to spell out the differences:

Age – The mid-life crisis is usually confined to the ages of 35 to 45, while andropause is characteristically 45 to 55, as with female menopause. However, if there was previous damage to the testes, such as from mumps, alcohol or vasectomy, andropause may arrive earlier.

Childhood – A disturbed, unsupportive childhood, one starved of love and affection, especially if accompanied by physical or mental abuse, is much more common in the background of someone experiencing a mid-life crisis.

Triggers – The death or serious illness of a parent or close friend is a common trigger of a mid-life crisis, as such events bring you face to face with your own mortality. They make you feel that you are next in the firing line, which in turn brings up thoughts and feelings about the meaning of your life and your past, present and future goals and achievements.[9]

Paradoxically, this crisis can come after a period of success even more often than after a dismal failure. It may even come when you find the love of your life, either in a person or an occupation, but feel that getting it is too late or an impossible dream. As 'crisis' suggests, it is decision time, but you agonize over the choices. You consider changing your job, your partner or your whole way of life. By contrast, andropause comes after redundancy, after heavy financial losses, after the business has failed or after divorce, rather than during the period leading up to them.

Relationships – The crisis is by its nature often very much about personal and business relationships. Questions about whether you want to continue living or working with someone, or staying in the same organization, are often uppermost in your mind. You think about them over and over, and may dream about them repeatedly at night.

During andropause, you are more likely to feel too weary to want to male any changes and too tired to even dream about doing so. Because of this lethargy, your marriage and business relationships may be falling apart around you, but you feel powerless to do anything about it.

Sex drive – This is most often increased during the crisis, either as a form of escapism, or as a conscious or subconscious way of bringing matters to a head. Sometimes, however, when a man is depressed by these events, as with other forms of depression, the libido may decrease. With andropause, the libido is almost always decreased, although occasionally there may be an affair to try to revive waning sexual powers.

Potency – There are few absolute rules about this, but aside from obvious physical causes such as diabetes, or the side effects of medicines to lower blood pressure or treat depression, or where triggered by severe psychosexual problems, only during andropause is potency consistently decreased over several months or years.

Physical symptoms – Fatigue, aches, pains and stiffness in the joints, night sweats and other physical symptoms which are typical of andropause are usually absent in mid-life crisis.

Hormone patterns – These are nearly always normal during the crisis, unless there is deep depression or heavy drinking. Although total testosterone is often normal during andropause, the free, biologically active testosterone typically is decreased, as described in the next chapter. There are also often other more subtle markers of this condition to confirm the diagnosis which can be found by careful and extensive hormone profiles of the blood.

Responses to treatment – Treatment of the crisis is mainly by counseling and support to help the person resolve the issues which are troubling him or her. Tranquilizers or antidepressants can occasionally be effective for short-term treatment if anxiety or depression is overwhelming. However they can be addictive and actually delay solving the problems which life has thrown up.

Testosterone will not help the person experiencing mid-life crisis but is likely to dramatically benefit those suffering the miseries of andropause.

Mid-Life Crisis Checklist (MLC)

To find out whether you yourself, a friend or a relative is going through the Male Mid-Life Crisis, check out the following questions:

1.	Age	30s	40s	50s	60s
2.	Death of Parent within	1 yr	2 yrs	3 yrs	4 yrs
3.	Death of Close Friend within	1 yr	2 yrs	3 yrs	4 yrs
4.	Change or Loss of Job within	1 yr	2 yrs	3 yrs	4 yrs
5.	Change or Loss of Partner within	1 yr	2 yrs	3 yrs	4 yrs
6.	Satisfaction with Present Partner	Bad	Poor	Fair	Good
7.	Satisfaction with Present Work	Bad	Poor	Fair	Good
8.	Satisfaction with your Childhood	Bad	Poor	Falr	Good
9.	Confidence about Role in Life	Bad	Poor	Fair	Good
10.	Sex Drive (Libido)	Good	Average	Fair	Bad
11.	Potency (Erections)	Good	Average	Fair	Bad
12.	Mental Energy	Good	Average	Fair	Bad
13.	Physical Energy	Good	Average	Fair	Bad

14. Creativity	Good	Average	Fair	Bad
15. Day Dreaming	Regular	Often	Seldom	None
16. Night Dreaming	Regular	Often	Seldom	None
17. Heavy Drinking	Regular	Often	Seldom	None
18. Tranquilizer Use	Regular	Often	Seldom	None
19. Thoughts about Dying	Regular	Often	Seldom	None
20. Thoughts about Major Life Changes	Regular	Often	Seldom	None

TOTAL CHECKS   ——   ——   ——   ——

Multiply checks in each column by: 3   2   1   0

TOTAL SCORES   ——   ——   ——   ——

TOTAL MID-LIFE CRISIS SCORE   ——

MID-LIFE CRISIS RATING: 0-9 UNLIKELY, 10-19 POSSIBLE, 20-29 LIKELY, 30-39 VERY LIKELY, 40+ SEVERE

The game of mid-life crisis survival

Like the name of the James Bond story, *You Only Live Twice*, for some men a second life really does begin at 40. For many, either on a plateau or steadily on the way up, this period may just be a natural continuation of the old life and they don't experience it as a crisis. For others there is a period of great unrest and inner turbulence, the 'Dark Night of the Soul,' but they come through it and either decide to climb up to fresh peaks or settle for a comfortable life in the valley. A few, unfortunately, get addicted to alcohol or drugs, sexual excess or risky behavior and may or may not survive the experience. Others lose their direction or fall prey to depression. Sometimes they find themselves and make successful changes in their lives, or sometimes their fortune changes.

Often this crisis takes place very publicly in showbusiness celebrities whose careers have taken off or whose unstable relationships have broken down. These events bring with them large-scale publicity which can lead to what has recently been described by British journalist A. A. Gill as 'over-exposure on the media mountain.' Stars who get sucked into this media circus can find they suddenly fall into obscurity or are buried under an avalanche of hype. Some never recover. Like the British comedian Tony Hancock, they may commit suicide, or, like Peter Sellers, drive themselves to heart attacks, which are often due to the inner enemies of anger and despair.[10]

Surviving the mid-life crisis

There is a great deal to learn from all these stories about how to come through your own mid-life crisis, if you are having one, or how to help other people through theirs.

Make a map

For the person who decides that they have reached mid-life, or those trying to help them, it helps to make a map. Where are you now and where, if anywhere, do you want to get to? Some people are destined to climb one peak of achievement or creativity, often in their twenties or thirties, and then plateau off at mid-life or go downhill. Others achieve a second, perhaps even higher peak later in life, having successfully dealt with their mid-life crisis using the experience, knowledge and wisdom built up in the first half of their lives. This can happen in all walks of life, but particularly with writers, who breathe in experience and breathe out prose, with applied scientists, and sometimes with businessmen, who may hit the financial rocks in mid-life, but learn important lessons and go on to rebuild their empires.

You need to decide what realistically are your goals and how worthwhile are they to you? How high do you want to climb? How much effort are you willing to put in and what risks are you willing to take? Are you content with what you have achieved and the part you have played in life so far? As the financier Bernie Cornfield, who created the huge financial bubble of Investors in Overseas Securities, IOS, or, as it could have been more accurately called, IOU, put it, 'Do you sincerely want to be rich?' Do you? Or do you have other priorities?

Resources for the journey

Having decided where you want to go, or at least the general direction, you need to make a full and fearless inventory of your resources in terms of health, finances and abilities. Don't forget to include the emotional support of your family and friends among your assets, as they can be crucial, especially if you are making radical changes to your life.

Also make a list of your weaknesses and the emotional baggage you are carrying. How much of it is necessary and how much can you leave behind you? How much 'unfinished business' do you have with a difficult childhood or family relationships? Could you finish it, if necessary with the help of a psychotherapist or analyst? What are your addictions, if any: alcohol, drugs, work, chocolate, food, sex? Think about where you can get help with these, because they can cripple you on the next part of your journey or even stop you ever getting started. What's your Achilles heel and how can you guard it?

In the final analysis you have to decide what you can change in yourself, as it has to be accepted that you can't change the world or others. If you decide you do wish, and are able, to make changes, probably the best idea is to follow the business tradition of making a five year plan to aid you in your journey and decide what you would like to have achieved by then. 'Realistic, but optimistic' is probably the best motto, but think carefully whether you will be able to live at peace with yourself and those around you if you realize your new ambition or continue with your old one.

If you think you can cope with or have coped with the hazards of a mid-life crisis, you may be interested in reducing your chances of experiencing andropause. The next chapter tells you how this happens and how your response to mid-life crisis may have either set you up for it or protected you from ever getting it.

Chapter four

How it happens

Why should one man in his forties or fifties suffer all the miseries of male menopause and another in his seventies or eighties escape them entirely? I am reminded of a cold, damp and miserable Viking warrior standing on a bleak landscape in a thunderstorm, shaking his fist at the sky and crying out, 'Why me, O Lord? Why me?' After pausing for thought, a thunderous voice from the heavens replies, 'Why not?'

Similarly, although the roots of this condition can usually be traced to one or several events, sometimes its causes remain unknown.

Let's look first at how testosterone is produced and its key role as a major contributor to the force that shapes our lives.

Hormone of kings – king of hormones

The hormone testosterone brings us into being. It regulates the sex drive in both men and women, it develops the male sexual characteristics such as dominance, drive, assertiveness, strength, body shape, hairiness and even odor in the form of pheromones. It governs sperm production as well as potency and therefore has the deciding vote on whether or not conception takes place.

It is a major factor in determining, both physically and mentally, whether we develop into a man or a woman, a homosexual or a heterosexual, a poet or a boxer, a wimp or a champ. As described in the book by Anne Moir and David Jesell, *Brain Sex: The real difference between men and women*,[1] testosterone literally shapes our brain and our creativity, intellectual skills, thought patterns, drive and determination to explore ideas and follow them through. It is an overriding influence in controlling not only our potential, but also the use we make of it. It governs our sexual and social history.

Testosterone also affects our health throughout life – how we grow as children, whether we thrive, whether we become a muscular Adonis in our teens or a beanpole with acne, even whether we are likely to die in a fight or motorcycle accident in our youth. It affects to what extent stress undermines our health in middle age and how we may die from the premature aging that its deficiency can cause. Ultimately it controls both our vitality and longevity.

As mentioned, testosterone can also be regarded as the 'success hormone.' A study funded by the National Institute of Health compared testosterone levels with personality type in more than 1,700 men. According to Dr John McKinlay, the medical statistician who analyzed the results, the male with high testosterone, the High-T Guy, *typically attempts to influence and control other people ... expresses his opinion forcibly and his anger freely, and ... dominates social interactions.* Having innately and persistently high levels of testosterone seems to make these men hard-driving, competitive and sometimes more successful.[2]

Once these patterns of behavior are established, lowering testosterone activity may cause them to fade, but treatment even with high doses of the hormone will only restore them to normal for that individual and not overshoot to cause aggression, antisocial activities or hyper-sexuality.

These findings closely mirrored those of Professor James Dabbs, a psychologist at Georgia State University. He studied 5,000 Vietnam War veterans and found that antisocial 'sensation seeking' behavior more often occurred in high-testosterone men with little education and low-income jobs. Those with more education and money had opportunities for a wider range of outlets for this type of behavior. 'They can do things that are both exciting and sociably acceptable – driving fast cars rather than stealing them, and arguing instead of fighting,' said Dabbs. He also found that men and women in more extrovert and expressive occupations – actors, entertainers, football players and even women lawyers – had high levels of testosterone, while clergymen had low levels. In this way it seems that testosterone affects every aspect of our lives as men.[3]

High-T Male Checklist (HTM)

These questions are designed to test whether you, a friend or a partner, are or were, a 'High Testosterone Male,' the type who only feels and functions well when their testosterone levels are high.

If the score is high on this test, **as rated from the overall life history**, it does not mean that testosterone levels are still high, as these men may be more liable to experience the symptoms of a shortage of this hormone, either male menopause or **andropause**.

Rate each of the following by selecting a value of 0-4 to represent the range from none or not at all = 0, slight = 1, moderate = 2, severe = 3, to extreme = 4.

	0	1	2	3	4
1. A leader in the type of work	—	—	—	—	—
2. Competitive	—	—	—	—	—
3. Power job, eg Lawyer, MD, CEO, politician	—	—	—	—	—
4. Energetic	—	—	—	—	—
5. High earner	—	—	—	—	—
6. Risk taker	—	—	—	—	—
7. A winner	—	—	—	—	—
8. Early and intense puberty	—	—	—	—	—
9. Acne as a teenager or later	—	—	—	—	—
10. Hairy chest, arms or legs	—	—	—	—	—
11. Athletic/Muscular	—	—	—	—	—
12. Highly sexed as a young man	—	—	—	—	—
13. Multiple sexual relationships	—	—	—	—	—
14. Alcohol related problems	—	—	—	—	—
15. Male relatives rating highly on the above scores	—	—	—	—	—
TOTALS	—	—	—	—	—

TOTAL HTM SCORE ___

HIGH-TESTOSTERONE RATING: 0-15 Unlikely, 16-30 Possible, 31-45 Likely, 46-60 Highly Likely, 61+ Extremely High-T.

Testosterone production

The command center for testosterone control is the brain. This has a variety of interrelated checks and balances which promote or suppress production, according to the needs of the body at a particular stage and time in life.

The most sophisticated part of the brain, the cerebral cortex, stimulates testosterone production when we are aroused and feeling successful in life. When we feel bored, angry, overstressed and losing life's battles, our testosterone goes down. These reactions are controlled each day by the hypothalamus, the 'impresario' at the base of the brain, and each hour by the pituitary gland, the 'conductor of the hormone orchestra of the body.' In adults this vital gland is the size and shape of a small cherry and suspended by a short stalk from the hypothalamus, from which it receives its regulatory messages. Accordingly, it produces a wide variety of key hormones which stimulate or suppress the various glands in the body, including the testes.

The pituitary hormones which control the sexual organs in both men and women are called gonadotrophins. There are two of these, named according to their functions in the female. One is called follicle stimulating hormone (FSH), because it stimulates the growth of follicles in the ovary which contain the eggs. In men it is mainly concerned with promoting sperm production. The other is called luteinizing hormone (LH); it regulates the production of estrogen by the ovaries and testosterone by the testes. Recent research suggests however that there are some interactions between these hormones in controlling testosterone production.[4]

Research has shown that over 95 percent of the 6-7 mg of the testosterone produced daily by the young male comes from the 500 million 'Leydig' cells in the testes; the remaining 5 per cent comes from the adrenal glands capping both kidneys. Blood testosterone levels in men are usually 10 to 20 times more than those in women, where the adrenals and ovaries are the main production sites. Eunuchs are therefore likely to have the same testosterone levels as women, just as men usually have the same estrogen levels as post-menopausal women whose ovaries have stopped its production.

Cholesterol is the raw material from which testosterone is synthesized in the body. In 1984, a group of Finnish researchers showed that low fat diets, especially when the proportion of the 'healthy' unsaturated fats was increased, lowered both total and free testosterone levels in the blood. This may be one explanation for the sad fact that any decrease in heart disease produced by these diets or cholesterol-lowering drugs tends to be outweighed by increased deaths from suicide, homicide and accidents, some of which might be linked to testosterone-deficient andropausal mood changes.[5]

It seems unfair that the 'rabbit food' diet foisted on an unsuspecting public by dietary dogmatists might be contributing to lower testosterone activity and the apparently increased level of erection problems in men. One wonders what the more drastic cholesterol lowering drugs are doing to the androgen levels of some of my patients who were put on them just before the onset of andropausal symptoms.

On the other hand, we have the sexually athletic performances of the legendary sixteenth century lover Giacomo Casanova, who boosted his testosterone levels with large numbers of raw eggs before each of his amorous marathons. It was reputedly the pox rather than heart disease which killed him at the age of 73.

Also, as pointed out in my book, *The Western Way of Death: Stress, tension and heart disease,*[6] 75 per cent of the cholesterol circulating in the bloodstream is made by the liver and increased by stress, whereas only 25 per cent comes from diet. Stress has other harmful effects, such as raising blood pressure and increasing blood clotting. So there is a lot of evidence that where heart disease is concerned, *'It's not so much a matter of what you eat as what's eating you.'*

One of the many compounds produced on the long production line from cholesterol to testosterone rejoices in the name of dehydroepiandrosterone, known to its aficionados as DHEA. This is an interesting steroid because its production rate is directly related to that of testosterone. It has also been shown to decrease with age, which offers further evidence about the possible origin of andropause. Given to aging men by Dr Etienne-Emil Baulieu in a clinical trial at the Institute of Health and Medical Research in Paris, it provided some of the benefits of testosterone treatment. However, DHEA is more expensive than testosterone and seems a roundabout way of promoting its synthesis, if that is what is needed. Also, some may be converted into estrogen, which antagonizes testosterone actions and so, in certain patients it could be counterproductive. However it is certainly worth looking further at it as a way of increasing natural testosterone production in the body.

Similarly a hormone from the pituitary gland, growth hormone, can boost the action of testosterone and has been claimed to have rejuvenated a small number of veterans on whom it was tried.[7] However, it required twice weekly injections, was about 10 times as expensive as testosterone and unlike that very safe medication, raised blood pressure and sugar levels.

Testosterone throughout life

Even in the womb, there are larger amounts of testosterone in the blood of males than females. This starts as early as six weeks after conception, reaches a peak of five to six times higher at 23 weeks, and then returns to female levels at about six months of intra-uterine life. By that time, of course, development of all the organs in the body is nearly complete, and the male or female die is cast.

Testosterone largely controls the development of the penis and the descent of the testes into the scrotum prepared to receive them. It also affects the brain, where the balance in function between the two hemispheres is supposed to be influenced by this hormonal difference. The mountain of inescapable evidence that men are different from women in a whole range of aptitudes, skills and abilities, and that these differences depend much more on hormonal nature than social nurture, is brilliantly reviewed in *Brain Sex*.[1]

After birth there is another surge of testosterone in the male, going up almost to adult male levels. It starts at about two weeks, reaches a peak at 10 weeks and then drops back to female levels at six months and stays there until puberty. These early months are also a period of active brain growth and development during which further sexual differentiation can arise. It seems likely that the traumas of birth and the first six months of life, such as prematurity, failure of maternal bonding, malnutrition and infections, might all reduce testosterone production and be factors which predispose a sickly infant to be a sickly adult.

At puberty in the male, testosterone levels rise rapidly, reaching a maximum of about 20 to 30 times the infant level at about age 18. This causes the pubertal development of hair on the face, armpits, pubes and, to a more variable extent, mainly due to hereditary factors, the rest of the body. Whether a man goes bald or not later in life again seems to be down more to heredity than hormones, unless he is castrated before puberty. It's what's in his genes that decides whether he keeps his hair for life, rather than what's in his jeans.

Also at puberty, the testes enlarge and descend into the scrotum, libido surges, the penis enlarges, erections occur spontaneously, particularly at night and in the early morning, and if not relieved by masturbation or intercourse, spontaneous emissions or 'wet dreams' happen, all of which can be associated with an unreasonable amount of adolescent emotional upset and guilt. At the same time the voice tone deepens and 'breaks,' due to thickening of the vocal cords, and the excess hormones and the pheromones are poured out in the sweat and skin oil, the sebum, which causes the social and physical discomforts of acne. Helped by growth hormone from the pituitary gland, there is an increase in muscle and bone growth in the male, but above a certain level testosterone switches off the latter, and between the ages of 18 and 20 growth usually ceases.

In eunuchs, and men who have low levels of testosterone because the testes fail to develop or descend, growth may continue and the man gets taller than other men in his family. At the other extreme, high levels of testosterone may arrest bone growth, and a highly sexed and hairy, shorter man will result. This could be the hormonal history of cuddly Dudley Moore, once described as a 'sex-thimble,' and the far less cuddly but also sexually active Napoleon Bonaparte. The statue of him (Napoleon, that is, not Dudley) standing naked in heroic pose on show in Apsley House at Hyde Park Corner in London indicates that he was well endowed in sexual structure as well as function. However, by the time he died, a beaten man possibly suffering lead poisoning, Napoleon was found to have severe genital atrophy. Wonderful are the permutations and combinations of heredity, hormones and history which produce the individual physique and temperament.

Testosterone and male menopause

One of the main reasons why the idea of male menopause has proved so controversial is that unlike female menopause, where there is a clear and easily measurable precipitous drop in estrogen level, it is difficult to show any such fall in males suffering similar symptoms. To understand why this is so, we must enterprisingly 'boldly go' a little deeper into the mechanics of testosterone control and action.

The small but vital amounts of testosterone produced in the testes are immediately swept away around the body in the bloodstream and are mainly bound to a special carrier protein called sex hormone binding globulin. This SHBG, as it is usually called, is a key player in this 'Who stole the testosterone?' mystery, since it grabs the hormone and runs, and seems reluctant to part with it. The more SHBG there is, the less free, active, 'bio-available' testosterone is able to get out of the blood into the cells to do its job.

The availability of the testosterone can be measured as the 'free androgen index,' or FAI, which is the total testosterone level in the blood divided by the SHBG level multiplied by 100, and is normally between 70 and 100 per cent in young men. It is when the FAI falls below 50 per cent that symptoms of andropause usually appear. This has been one of the key findings in my research.

The way in which the body regulates the amount of testosterone available at any one time works well in youth, when there is usually plenty of testosterone and its level of activity is controlled by a roughly equivalent amount of SHBG. If testosterone levels drop temporarily for any reason, the SHBG falls to compensate for this, and so the amount of testosterone available, expressed by the FAI, is kept constant. However, later in life, especially around the age of 50, this 'testostat' mechanism often seems to break down and andropause results. A car dealer patient of mine called SHBG, 'Sex Hand-Brake Globulin,' because he felt his hormonal engine was revving, but his brakes were on.

What goes wrong in this key part of the body's hormonal balance? There are two possible explanations. The first is that the amount of testosterone 'income' falls due to understimulation of the testes by the hypothalamus and pituitary, a deficiency of raw materials for its production and wearing out of the testes. The second is that the 'expenditure' rises, in terms of amount of testosterone taken up by the SHBG and that used up in repairing the ravages of age, stress, alcohol and other forms of wear and tear. Also, the cells all over the body which are targets for Cupid's testosterone arrows may become tougher with age, more difficult to penetrate and less responsive to its effects.

A life-long program of research by a Belgian professor, Alex Vermeulen at the University of Ghent, has shown that all stages in the production and action of testosterone can be affected by the aging process.[8] The amount of testosterone that is produced falls particularly after middle age because of aging of the interstitial cells that produce it in the testes. In the 1960s, this process was made very clear because the amount of testosterone appearing in the urine was found to drop steadily with age, since it represents the 'free', active hormone.[9] Other doctors have shown that from about the age of 40 onward, testicular size and the amount of free testosterone begins to decrease, and the pituitary driving force increases to try and compensate.[10]

However, what still confuses critics of male menopause theory even today is that the level of total testosterone as measured in the blood only falls slightly up to age 70. This is because the hormone is being held in the blood by rising levels of SHBG and so less is 'bio-available' to be taken up by the target receptors in the tissues or excreted in the urine.[11,12]. This has been confirmed in the first 400 of my male menopause patients, where only 13 per cent showed abnormally low total testosterone levels in the blood, but, mainly because of raised SHBG levels, about 75 percent had a low free androgen index. About 70 percent also showed raised levels of the pituitary gonadotrophin hormones which stimulate the testis, the LH and FSH, which confirms that the level of testosterone activity is insufficient for the body's needs.

As already mentioned, this situation was recognized and proved from urinary studies in the 1940s, but thanks to the complications introduced by blood tests, doctors are still able to argue about it to this day. Many patients have come to me saying that they had classic andropausal symptoms, but their doctors measured their total testosterone level, found it normal or low normal, and said that there was nothing wrong with their hormones and the problem must all be psychological. Fortunately some patients persevere in the belief that it is their hormones that are out of order rather than their minds, get the additional tests done to complete the diagnosis and start testosterone treatment.

Early disturbances

The normal patterns in hormonal development can be delayed, arrested or modified at any stage of life. About 10 percent of male menopause patients I have seen probably had lower than normal testosterone levels from puberty onward. These cases were sometimes due to the testes never having functioned properly because they failed to descend into the scrotum, only partially descended, or retracted back into the abdomen too easily.

These varying degrees of partial nonfunctioning or impaired development of the testis may not be obvious, or indeed interfere (noticeably) with sexual characteristics or function until middle age or later.

The estrogen threat to the male

As well as the decreasing amounts and activity of testosterone, the threat to male fertility and virility can be explained by increasing exposure to xeno-estrogens, chemicals in the environment with actions similar to those of the female hormone estrogen, and to anti-androgens, which have recently been found to have an anti-testosterone action.[13,14]

Estrogens, although essential for the development of female characteristics, seem to work against the actions of testosterone in the male. Derived from everything from plastics to pesticides, they are thought to be having a harmful effect on fertility and the sexual development of male offspring, and even to be contributing to rising testicular and prostate cancer rates. Their effect was seen most dramatically in women given the strong synthetic estrogen stilboestrol during pregnancy to reduce the changes of a miscarriage. When their sons were born, a considerable number had undescended testes and abnormal genital development. Later in life they were also found to be infertile because of low sperm counts.

For a wide and increasing variety of reasons men seem to be drowning in a sea of estrogens. Even the uterine bath water they swim in during the first nine months of life is laced with rising levels of hormonally-active compounds. Evidence of this is the increasing number of boys being born with hormonally caused birth defects in their sexual characteristics. This is especially marked in the condition known as hypospadias, where the penis is poorly developed and opens towards the base rather than at the tip. Also, because of the continuing influence of these estrogenic compounds, the testes increasingly often fail to descend from the abdomen into the scrotum, which not only decreases their ability to produce sperm, but also reduces their testosterone producing capacity.[15]

Perhaps future generations of archeologists will come across thick layers of plastic bags, marking the demise of *homo plasticus* or 'plastic bag man' who was neutered by the by-products of the consumer society.

Exposure to estrogens at any time of life can have a bad effect in the male, but particularly around the time of puberty. One patient of mine, when at college in his late teens, made the mistake of telling his college doctor that he felt over-sexed. The doctor overreacted by giving him a month's course of estrogen. It worked – his libido died overnight and he was able to concentrate on his studies. The unfortunate thing was that his libido never recovered, he never married or had children, and when he came to see me at the age of 45 it seemed that he had premature andropause, with no other apparent cause than the estrogen.

An interesting subgroup of my patients made up of farmers, appeared to show occupational risk factors for andropause. The health of these 'front-line' troops in the agrochemical arms race towards greater productivity and profitability makes an interesting study in relation to chemical pollution of the environment.[16]

In some, the causative agent of their symptoms appeared obvious. The main relevant feature of their case histories was that they had worked on farms when they were young men caponizing chickens or turkeys with estrogen pellet implants or creams to make the birds plumper and more tender. Unfortunately, although it might be considered poetic justice, they must have taken in large amounts of estrogen themselves, either by absorption through the skin or lungs, or by eating the birds shortly after the treatment, which caused them to become caponized themselves.

In a similar case concerning cattle, an andropausal patient from Canada recently told me how he and his brother often ate beef raised on his farm often without waiting for the 48-hour so-called safety limit to expire, after giving their cattle long-acting hormone cocktails designed to promote growth for up to three months. Either they misread the instructions or they were being seriously misled by the manufacturers of these dollar-a-shot mixtures.

In addition to severe andropausal symptoms of fatigue, depression, irritability and loss of libido and potency, these farmworkers often showed enlargement of their breasts (gynecomastia), testicular atrophy, low total testosterone, high SHBG giving a reduced free androgen index, and elevated FSH and LH levels.

Another subgroup of farmers, however, had similar symptoms, but with a history of exposure to other potentially antitestosterone hormones or pesticides used in farming. Here the clinical and endocrine features were less marked. Fortunately both groups responded well to androgen treatment, either orally or by testosterone pellet implant.

The latter group, however, could well have been an example of antiandrogen activity from any one of a wide range of antimicrobial agents, pesticides and fungicides. For example, it was observed in 1971 that coccidiostats that were given to chickens produced maximum weight gain for minimum food intake, but they were banned because they caused men to develop large womanly breasts and become infertile.

A wide range of drugs used in medicine are known to have this property. Detailed studies of such compounds, taking into account the possibly differing effects of different forms of the same molecule (stereo-isomers), may give clues to their complex hormonal interactions.

My first Professor of Biochemistry at the Middlesex Hospital in London, Sir Charles Dodds, who was working with a group in Oxford, was the first to describe xeno-estrogens in an article in *Nature* dated February 5 1938: 'The Estrogenic Activity of Certain Synthetic Compounds.' He compared the structure of what he proposed should be called 'stilbestrol,' which his group had just synthesized, with the naturally occurring hormone called estrone.[17]

Later the same year he described the estrogenic actions of a range of related compounds and noted the 'large effects of relatively small changes' in related molecules.[18] These two historic papers set the scene for mass production of estrogenic compounds for both therapeutic and veterinary purposes, and could explain some of our present concerns on the effects of xeno-estrogens and androgen receptor antagonists.

Just as small changes in molecules can greatly increase their estrogen activity, so apparently minor modifications can make them much more powerful antiandrogens. This was dramatically demonstrated by

Kelce and his co-workers in an article in *Nature* in 1995 which showed how the major and persistent metabolite of DDT, *p.p.*-DDE, had little estrogenic activity, but 15 times the antiandrogen effect of the parent compound.[19]

This was one-fifth of the potency, if that is the right word, of flutamide, the most powerful antiandrogen used in medical and veterinary practice, with the well-known side effects of severe andropausal symptoms and gynecomastia. The similarities in the structural formulas of these compounds, along with the antiandrogen vinclozolin, which is used in agriculture as a fungicide, are apparent when you look at their molecular structure.

Fortunately, the chemical castration in animals and humans by the use of overtly estrogenic compounds in veterinary practice was banned in the UK in 1986 and in the remainder of the European Union by a hormonal growth promoter ban in 1988. However the practice still continues secretly in some countries, along with the dangerous business of giving a range of chemical cocktails to farmyard animals to improve the amount and texture of meat, or more recently their milk yield, by using genetically engineered bovine somatotrophin (rBST).

In the USA and Canada, hormones are more widely used in meat production and the European Union is under increasing pressure from the World Trade Organization (WTO) to take more hormonally treated meat from these countries.

The effects on estrogen and androgen receptors of a wide range of products used in veterinary medicine and agriculture should be investigated urgently, and any of the commercial pressures to reverse the EU ban on hormonal growth promoters should be resisted until research has proven them safe for human health.

It took 50 years to learn the lesson spelled out by Sir Charles Dodds in 1938 and ban estrogenic substances from veterinary practice, but now apparently, we have the itch to unlearn it. Should we be going 'back to nature' to learn the 1995 message from Kelce and his co-workers about the possible antiandrogenic effects of a wide range of agrochemicals?

Viral and bacterial infections

Infections can also be linked to testicular damage. Two thousand years Hippocrates recognized that mumps sometimes caused shrinkage of the testicles and infertility later in life. In general, anything which affects fertility in the male is also likely to influence testosterone production. However the medical profession often does not appreciate how a long-forgotten childhood illness can contribute to precipitating andropause 30 or 40 years later.

The testis seems liable to be damaged by the mumps virus, and perhaps other viruses, only from the first stirrings of puberty onward. This seems to be because of the intense activity, cell division and growth in the testis during this time.

Before the age of 10 or 12, mumps is a highly infectious viral illness passed from child to child, causing a mild fever and the very characteristic swelling of the parotid salivary glands in front of both ears, which usually passes without complications within a few days. An attack of mumps at this age is usually entirely harmless and gives valuable immunity which frequently lasts for life.

If a man picks up the infection at any time beyond this age, however, he is likely to be more ill and one or both testes may become very painful, swollen and inflamed, a condition known as orchitis. This very uncomfortable condition, sometimes described by the song title 'Great Balls of Fire,' can last one or two weeks or even longer. It then subsides, often leaving scarring of one or both testes, which may be shown by shrinkage or softening.[20]

Infertility after mumps is fortunately uncommon, but in many cases there may be damage to the testosterone producing cells which becomes apparent later in life. Eleven percent of my andropause patients reported a history of mumps after the age of 12 and in these cases, which tended to be the younger patients, there was often no other obvious cause. These are good reasons why more boys should be immunized early in infancy.

Although mumps is by far the most obvious and common virus attacking the testis, there is some evidence that a wide range of other viruses may sometimes be involved. However, because the orchitis is a less prominent feature of a generalized feverish illness that makes the patient feel rotten all over, their influence may be overlooked.

Again, it is probably when the testis is most active, around the age of puberty, that it is most susceptible to damage by viruses.

Another virus which has been definitely recorded as occasionally causing orchitis is glandular fever, also known as infectious mononucleosis or the 'kissing disease,' as outbreaks seemed to spread among boys and girls in this way, although this could just be parental propaganada.[21]

Sometimes patients date their andropausal symptoms from some unidentified viral illness, although whether this directly affected their testosterone production or was just the last straw that caused a hormonal breakdown is unclear. The fatigue, depression and loss of libido that accompanies many viral conditions, especially myalgic encephalitis (ME), can mimic many of the symptoms of male menopause, and careful history taking and hormonal tests are needed to distinguish between them. Similarly, the general malaise affecting patients during a severe attack of jaundice, whether due to hepatitis A, B or the newly discovered insidious variety C, is likely to reduce the patients' testosterone production, whether the testes are directly affected or not.

Other infections of the testes and prostate also seem liable to affect testosterone levels. Both so-called 'non-specific urethritis,' a common cause of penile soreness and discharge, and the better known sexually transmitted diseases such as syphilis or gonorrhea can cause a reduction in testosterone. Sometimes infections of the prostate and testis can also occur after surgery to the prostate or bladder, with the same result.

The possible involvement of so many infections in contributing to male menopause underlines the need for doctors involved in its treatment to take a full case history. Much further research is needed to see which infections, at what age, need to be avoided or treated to maintain full testicular function.

Stress

Men under stress exhibit lack of sexual desire and performance, particularly when they grow older. Younger men, especially those going through male mid-life crisis, may use sex as a means of relieving tension or trying to restore confidence, but over the age of 50 the stressed male is more likely to just stop trying. This is a natural biological reaction and is seen throughout the animal kingdom.

In over half the men in my clinic, stress assessed as excessive 'life events' appeared to be the factor which precipitated andropause. This was much more evident with the stresses of failure and defeat in life's battles than those of success. Divorce, insolvency, heavy financial losses, unemployment, recession in business and losing court cases were all big put downs, mentally and then physically. Conversely, successful remarriage, the start of a new relationship, getting a desired job or promotion or winning the lottery could fan the flames, or sometimes even the ashes, of both virility and vitality. Even a good relaxing holiday can sometimes have the same effect, although all too often the benefits fade as rapidly as a suntan when the man returns to his stressful workaday world.

Why does stress have such a powerful effect on people's sex lives? Obviously it is partly a direct psychological effect. If the brain, which has been described as the biggest sex organ in the body, is directing its attentions mainly towards survival in the urban jungle, sexual activity will have a low priority.

Anxiety, too, is a definite turn off, and performance anxiety, as we have seen, can be a self-fulfilling prophesy.

Excessive stress – 'stress overload' – can also act by reducing testosterone levels. This has been shown by research studies into a wide variety of situations carried out since the 1960s.[22] One of the first of these was a study into the stress of airline travel that I made with an Argentinean doctor, Emil Arguelles.[23] He was able to show that exposing young men working in a factory to a couple of hours of air-turbine noise was enough to halve their blood testosterone levels. He had already shown lowered testosterone in men following heart attacks.[24]

Moderately stressful events, such as taking exams in an army officer cadet training school, could also lower testosterone levels, although this was less pronounced in successful candidates.[25]

Even experiencing less intense stress, such as losing $100 in a tennis match, was enough to cause a noticeable drop in testosterone.[26] While mild to moderately intense physical stress, including intercourse, seems to increase testosterone levels, severe exertion such as running marathons was found to lower them.[27,28]

A final action of stress is to cause the release of 'stress hormones' such as adrenaline, noradrenaline and cortisol. These are breakdown 'catabolic hormones' which work against the build-up of 'anabolic hormones,' principally testosterone. The former raise blood sugar and fat levels and increase oxygen consumption, while the latter have the opposite action.

Alcohol

Shakespeare, in *Macbeth*, describes drink as provoking desire, but taking away performance. This is one of the common ways in which erectile problems associated with andropause first begin to show during middle age.

This contrasts with women, who are more susceptible to the effects of alcohol than men and yet are more sexually stimulated by it. Recent research in Sweden showed that three glasses of wine rapidly raised testosterone levels in girls in their twenties, more than in a group of men the same age. This combination of a lessening of inhibitions and an increase in the hormone which stimulates the libido, explains the old saying, 'Candy is dandy, but liquor is quicker.' However, many women also find that it is more difficult to have an orgasm when drunk.

It is surprising how strong a poison to the testis alcohol is. It may act directly or through its immediate breakdown product, acetaldehyde[29] or by increasing SHBG.[30] Either way, even in moderate drinkers, blood testosterone levels fall as alcohol levels increase. Drinking enough to cause a hangover has been found to lower testosterone levels 12 to 20 hours later – in one study to 20 percent of their levels before drinking. Perhaps sagging hormone levels are one of the reasons why a hangover feels so awful. This might explain those eye-opening hangover cures such as 'Prairie Oyster,' based on boosting cholesterol levels with raw eggs.

This makes it less surprising that later in life, both because of long-term testicular damage and its short-term action in reducing testosterone levels and erectile function, alcohol can take away both desire and performance in men. Thirty percent of my first 1,000 andropausal patients reported drinking more than 21 units of alcohol a week and many drank two, three or four times that amount. (One unit equals a half pint of beer, a glass of wine or a measure of spirit.)

Although several studies have suggested that it's safe to drink up to 40 units of alcohol a week, especially as red wine may protect the heart through antioxidant and anti-coagulant effects, from the sexual function point of view alcohol is generally bad news both in the short and long term. Beer and lagers appear to be particularly toxic to the testis because they contain plant estrogens, called phyto-estrogens, from the hops, and other ingredients used in their production. Even low alcohol lagers and other drinks might contain these estrogens, and more research is needed on their effects.

A sixteenth-century Italian physician called Cornaro wrote, 'The excesses of our youth are like drafts upon our old age, payable with interest about twenty years after date.'[31] This is certainly true in relation to alcohol. As well as those andropausal patients who were drinking too much, about another 10 percent gave a past history of excess alcohol consumption for over a year or more. Unfortunately, testicular function does not seem to improve very much even if they subsequently stop drinking for several years.

This is in contrast to smoking, where most of the hazards, such as lung cancer and heart disease, decrease dramatically within five to ten years of giving up. The testis lacks the power of the liver to regenerate and never fully recovers, as is shown by the infertility, impotence and loss of libido that chronic alcoholics experience, even after drying out. The liver forgives and forgets, but the testis harbors grudges, so the bar-room bruisers of today are likely to be the lousy lovers of tomorrow.

The sensitivity of the testis to alcohol was clearly shown in recent studies conducted by a research group in Milan, Italy. They found that compared to nondrinkers, those who drank 14-21 units of alcohol per week were twice as likely to be subfertile and those who drank 28 units and over were nearly four times more likely. This factor is well recognized in infertility clinics, particularly as a cause of poor sperm motility. It seems that unlike the men who make them, sperm just don't drink and drive.

Overheating

The scrotum is not a design fault by our creator to use up spare skin, as the Scottish comedian Billy Connolly insists. Nature does not risk putting vital and sensitive glands in such an exposed position without an excellent reason. This is because to function properly they need to be a few crucial degrees cooler than the rest of the body. It's as though the testis has to pluck up the courage to make a small step outside the body into the cooler scrotum and testosterone drives it to do so. This is truly a giant leap for mankind, because unless it happens, neither the desire nor the ability to father children develop. As has been mentioned previously, the effect of xeno-estrogens to antagonize testosterone production and action may have contributed to the increased incidence of non-descent seen in recent years.

This temperature question can also cause problems during and after puberty when the scrotum is increasingly kept warm by jockey shorts and tight jeans. Together, these are likely to be as bad as the padded codpieces which reduced the fertility of Henry VIII and his courtiers. A condition called 'varicocele,' in which collections of fluid form in the scrotum and cause a warming, insulating effect, has also been shown to reduce testosterone levels, especially in older patients.[32]

There is an old country saying, 'Rams wrapped in wool breed no lambs.' This principle has been used by the Japanese, who have recently introduced a male contraceptive device consisting of a padded scrotal support. Worn continuously, it is said to be very effective in making men temporarily sterile after the 2-3 month period needed to allow sperm already produced to die off.

Even mental imaging techniques, as when some university students were asked to imagine warming of the scrotum as part of their system of autogenic mental exercises, are said to have produced a marked reduction in sperm count within a couple of months.

Other studies have suggested that the polyester component of underwear may generate electromagnetic fields which impair testicular function.

The importance of testicular cooling has recently received further scientific proof in an article in the *International Journal of Andrology* by a research group in Milan, where they know a thing or two about male fashion and its penalties. Infertility was nearly twice as common in men wearing tight underpants as men wearing loose boxer shorts, and one-and-a-half times as common in men wearing tight trousers, including jeans, as loose trousers. For men who combined the two and wore tight underpants and trousers, the risk of infertility was two-and-a-half times that of those who did neither.[33]

Perhaps this principle was recognized in the past. Loose-fitting underpants made of a leather cloth soft enough not to chafe the skin were worn by Viking warriors when invading Britain 3,000 years ago, according to a recent archeological find. However, the extremes of this advice to 'stay cool and hang loose,' were seen in the soldiers of the Black Watch Highland Regiment, who were forbidden to wear anything under their kilts. To enter or leave the barracks they had to walk over mirrors in the guard house, with their privates on parade, so to speak, to make sure they were obeying orders.

As testosterone production and sperm production appear, not surprisingly, to be closely linked, it seems the best way to promote virility as well as fertility is to recommend large, loose-fitting, lightweight cotton or silk boxer shorts. Perhaps 'Burn your bikinis' might be a good motto for 'men's lib.'

This explanation of the many ways in which the body's supplies of testosterone may be reduced or inactivated would be incomplete without a chapter on the important part unwittingly played by doctors themselves – vasectomy.

Chapter five

Vasectomy: The unkindest cut of all

The idea that vasectomy could be a major cause of andropause makes the many doctors who recommend it and those who inflict it on unsuspecting patients rush to its defense. Such reactions come with faith, but usually little detailed knowledge of the many possible adverse reactions to the operation.

Since vasectomy first came into fashion in the 1960s, this seemingly trivial operation has been described as anything from 'the most loving thing that a man can do for a woman' to 'the unkindest cut of all' – a 'surgical sword of Damocles' threatening the testes. Despite the controversy, it has really taken off as a means of contraception, and it is estimated that 500,000 Americans, 20,000 British, and 10,000 Irish men have it each year.

The first human vasectomy was performed in 1894 by a British surgeon to reduce the size of an enlarged prostate, which it apparently failed to do.[1] However, the operation did not become widespread until 1916, when a Viennese surgeon, Ludwig Steinach, proclaimed it as a method of rejuvenating the male. His theory was that if the part of the testicular factory manufacturing sperm were shut down, it would leave more room for the testosterone producing cells to flourish, which would reduce aging. The idea proved popular and on the basis of many reports from patients who claimed the operations had done wanders for them, thousands of men were 'Steinachered.' There were even reports that the illustrious father of psychoanalysis, Sigmund Freud, who also lived in Vienna, underwent the operation to promote longevity and revive his sexual powers – but perhaps this was just to overcome a psychological block.

From 1909 onwards, it was also used as a tool in social engineering, to limit reproduction by any people considered 'defective individuals.' A particular enthusiast for this form of eugenics was a Dr Harry Sharp, resident physician at the Jeffersonville Reformatory, Indiana. He compulsorily vasectomized 280 men because they had defects of character such as 'selfishness, ingratitude, inconstancy, egotism, and inability to resist any impulse or desire' or masturbated excessively. While these traits must obviously have been very rare in the population in those days, at least in Indiana, a considerable number might now be considered as eligible on these grounds in most countries.

People on whom this form of involuntary sterilization could be inflicted ranged from color-blind individuals to those considered undesirable because of their race or creed. From 1933 onwards, under the law 'Prevention of Hereditary Disease in Posterity,' the German government forced over a million men it considered unfit, including probably not coincidentally, a large proportion of Jewish people, to undergo vasectomy.

In the USA in 1922, 31 states had statues permitting involuntary sterilization of 'defective individuals.' Even with the outcry over its abuses by the Nazis, 21 states retained these laws after the Second World War, and as recently as 1973 Tennessee, Mississippi, Ohio and Illinois introduced bills ordering the sterilization of those on welfare with two or more children. California and Oklahoma made vasectomy a condition of suspending prison sentences in those convicted of robbery or not supporting their families.[2] In Britain the Child Support Agency seems to prefer financial castration.

In India, vasectomy has been vigorously promoted as a part of Government population policy. A new world record was achieved in 1971 by holding a 'Vasectomy Camp' which sterilized 63,000 men in one month. A hundred surgeons worked nonstop around the clock, while a variety of circus sideshows entertained those waiting their turn. Three years later it was revealed that gangs of 'motivators' who had been offered small sums to encourage men to undergo the operation, had misled or forcibly pressed or blackmailed them, and nearly half the men wished they had never had it done.[3]

In Britain in 1994 an alarming increase in vasectomy rates in men in their early twenties was thought to be due to the recession and job losses making it difficult to afford the cost of housing a family. One wonders how many of these men now regret the decision.

My first experience of the clinical effects of vasectomy was in 1979 when I first visited the clinic of Dr Jens Møller in Copenhagen. A surprising number of his patients – most of whom were being treated with testosterone for severe problems with the circulation in their legs, and often heart disease as well, had had a vasectomy many years before. When I commented on this, Dr Møller simply said, *'Ah yes. When I hear a patient has had a vasectomy, I know he is a case for me!'* This seemed at the time to be a rather extreme remark to make, but it prompted me to look up the literature on the subject.

Rather to my surprise, I found that there was a considerable amount of evidence to support Dr Møller's view that vasectomy might have harmful effects on the heart and circulation. I had not expected this, because it was such a commonly accepted operation and one which I had only just escaped having myself, in the nick of time, so to speak. It had been sold to the unsuspecting public, as it is still, as a snip. This stands for Simply No Immediate Problems. I pointed out in 1979 that this is a falsely simplistic view of a complex and important issue.[4]

Let's look first at what happens during and after the operation, and then at what can and does go wrong.

Unlike any other operation, however minor, no general medical examination is done beforehand, no central records are kept of how many operations have been performed and counseling is limited to telling the patient that it is irreversible so be sure you want it done. No inquiries are made into any previous history of mumps or other infections which may damage the testes, or of relevant family histories of heart disease, high blood pressure or diabetes. Any questions about what happens to the sperm are brushed aside with facile answers such as 'It is just absorbed.'

In order for patients to make an informed decision about whether to take a drug, it has to include in the packaging a formidable list of every complication, however rare, ever recorded in association with the use of that compound, and often for good measure with every related compound. The same should apply when an operation such as vasectomy is prescribed, but the possible complications discussed here are rarely mentioned and certainly not covered in the detail it deserves. Vasectomy is, after all, a major surgical insult to a very sensitive, delicate and highly tuned organ.

Vasectomy is a deceptively simple 'minor' operation and can be, and often is, carried out by the most junior and inexperienced of surgeons. It takes 15 minutes to one-half hour and so lends itself to mass application in clinics set up for the purpose on a conveyor belt system.[5]

The actual procedure is carried out under local anesthetic. Through a small incision, the tube carrying the sperm from the testis on each side to the prostate gland below the bladder, the *vas deferens* which gives the operation its name, is exposed. It is then dissected free of the fine nerves and blood vessels which run alongside it in the spermatic cord, and sealed off. This may be done by cutting it and tying off one or both ends, by frying it with electrocautery or by blocking it with a plastic spigot (this is claimed to be more easily reversible).

To the patient and surgeon alike it is seen as a simple plumbing job to turn off the stopcocks and prevent sperm getting out of the testes. It is presented as a cheap and effective form of contraception, for which one is awarded a portable radio for an act of social conscience in India and a tie inscribed IOFB, standing for '*I Only Fire Blanks,*' in Britain. (As the antivasection lobby gathers strength, refusenik members may well come to sport ties inscribed IOFLA, standing for '*I Only Fire Live Ammunition.*')

However, after the operation there may be a variety of complications, which can be divided into short and long term. The vas itself may be damaged, as can the fine blood vessels, nerves and lymph vessels which run alongside it in the spermatic cord. These nourish the testis, control its temperature to within very critical limits and drain fluid away from it. Temperature control of the testis can sometimes be impaired after vasectomy, along with fluid drainage from around it so that collections of fluid called hydrocele are formed in some cases. This insulating effect tends to raise the temperature, which can have a harmful effect on the testes' ability to produce both sperm and testosterone. Not only this, but there are also nerve connections between the two testes and damage to one can affect the other in a variety of ways.

There is often mild to moderate discomfort which may cause the patient to stay off work for anything from an hour to a week, depending on his pain threshold, motivation and how many of the fine nerve endings that run alongside the vas get caught up in the operation.

Fortunately quite infrequently, a variety of other changes can occur which cause a persistent and disabling 'post-vasectomy pain syndrome.'[6,7] If both ends of the vas have been tied off, the pressure in the stump attached to the testis builds up, and sometimes cysts form in the sperm-collecting tubules surrounding the testis. They can be felt as small lumps. Sometimes the cysts burst open and swellings at the severed ends of the vas arise called granulomas. They are due to a local tissue reaction to sperm. If the vas has been left open, then the sperm spills out into the loose tissue in the scrotum, and granulomas are then more likely to form than cysts.

In either case, but particularly where granulomas have formed, the body reacts to this highly unnatural no-exit situation by becoming allergic to its own sperm and producing anti-sperm antibodies. This is because sperm is only produced after puberty and is normally kept shielded from the body's immune system. The immune system would otherwise attack it, reacting just as it would to other 'alien' proteins such as those produced by bacteria and viruses. Vasectomy spills sperm into the tissues around the testis and exposes it to the antibody producing cells.[8]

You only have to meet a few patients with postvasectomy pain syndrome to be far more cautious about recommending the operation. One of these cases is Harry:

I had my vasectomy 10 years ago now and I haven't had a happy, painfree day since. It's been a nightmare from beginning to end and it's not over yet.

After seven years on the pill, my wife was advised to stop taking it and so I decided I'd have a vasectomy. On the day of the operation at our local hospital I had no second thoughts at all because I had heard that the procedure was quite straightforward. I was surprised therefore to wake from the general anesthetic with a tremendous pain in my stomach. The nurse reassured me the pain would go away and gave me valium. But when my friend arrived to take me home an hour later, I was still bent double with pain.

After a couple of days with no respite, I called in my own doctor who confirmed that it would settle down. But for the next few weeks I was only comfortable when I was lying down. Walking or lifting things was impossible and there was no question of being able to work. I was getting increasingly anxious as I had never really been ill before, but since both the hospital and my doctor were adamant there was nothing to worry about, I was prepared to give it time.

Then two months after the operation I found two small and painful lumps in each testicle. I was told these were sperm granulomas, the sperm not being properly absorbed into the body, and was shocked when the doctor told me he wasn't experienced in dealing with such problems and wanted to refer me to another hospital. By the time this appointment came up, the lumps had grown from being the size of match heads to the size of peas and they, together with the continuing ache in my stomach region, were causing me such discomfort that it was interfering with my whole life.

The new doctor performed an operation to remove the lumps. Afterwards he told me he believed too much of the vas had been cut away during the vasectomy, which explained the painful pulling sensation in my stomach, and I felt very angry. The lumps kept recurring and this was complicated by bouts of urinary infection that caused a painful inflammation in both testicles. To help this the surgeon finally had to remove the inflamed outer casting of the left testicle, the epididymis. Even this went wrong. Five months later the testis on that side began to shrink, and I had to have it removed and a plastic prosthesis put in.

By now I felt extremely low and tired and couldn't understand why. Some tests done down in London showed a very low testosterone level and that I was so allergic to my own sperm that even when they diluted my blood more than 20,000 times they could still get an anti-sperm reaction.

I was originally given some tablets called Proviron and these made me feel slightly better, although it took testosterone injections to make me feel much fitter. But even these wore off after a while. Last year I had to have the same series of operations on my right testicle, with removal of a granuloma, and then the epididymis, and now the testicle gets inflamed and is shrinking, so I may have to have even that removed.

It's been such a terrible time since the first operation. My job as a fork-lift truck driver, which I'd had for 18 years before the vasectomy, is gone, and my wife left me because it all got too much and we weren't having any fun or any sex. There have been times over the last few years when the pain and worry have made me think of ending it all, but things are slightly better now.

All this has been a result of a vasectomy that has gone wrong, probably because it was performed in a hurry by someone inexperienced, although I'm told it sometimes happens in the best of hands. This surgery sentenced me to 10 years' pain and misery.

Long-term complications of vasectomy my be much more common and diverse than is generally recognized. Of the limited amount of research which has been done, some is reassuring and some rather worrying.

Besides causing infertility problems in patients who want the vasectomy reversed, which happens in one percent of cases, no one seems to have thought through the other likely consequences. It's like tying a knot in the barrel of a rifle and being surprised when it blows back in your face!

I have been carrying out detailed antibody profiles in the post-vasectomy patients who have come to see me. There are some interesting but inconsistent findings which I am now analyzing in detail.

Some of my patients reported a prolonged and debilitating 'flu-like illness within the first few months after vasectomy, which is when immune reactions would be expected, and granulomas appear.

Some patients show an active generalized immune process as shown by raised levels in the blood of a protein called 'immune complement' which has been linked to the possibility of increased heart and circulatory disease after vasectomy.

The majority show anti-sperm antibodies. In fact it has been widely recognized and accepted for many years that anti-sperm antibodies are found in up to three-quarters of vasectomized men. One medical researcher on the subject cheerfully says, '*Vasectomy can be considered a particular form of experimental autoimmunization.*'[9]

An interesting, and as far as I know, unexplained sex difference is apparent here. When women develop anti-sperm antibodies, these usually cause the sperm to clump together 'head to head,' whereas the majority of my post-vasectomy men seem to have 'tail to tail' antibodies, sometimes active when their plasma is diluted over 16,000 times. Logic suggests that if you have antibodies against sperm, you might well develop antibodies against sperm-producing cells in the testis, the Sertoli or nurse cells, and indeed this is found in a proportion of cases.[10,11]

The discovery in other cases of antibodies against the testosterone producing, interstitial cells was unexpected, although this again seems logical. The sperm and testosterone producing cells work together, literally side by side, on the common mission of producing and launching these 'egg-seeking missiles.' Recent research has shown just how closely these functions are linked in many ways, including their own hormonal communications, the so-called paracrine actions.[12] If you suddenly shut one half of the factory, common sense would indicate that you might have some effect on the other. From my research and that of others, including testicular biopsies from vasectomized men, there is evidence that this is indeed the case.

Vasectomy and andropause

Over the last 10 years, I have been impressed by the fact that nearly 250 out of the 1,000 men in my initial research series complaining of symptoms of andropause have had vasectomies.

It is difficult to get accurate reports on the proportion of men in different countries who have had vasectomies, because the operation is assumed safe and thought too trivial to be worth recording. However, as the best estimate of the frequency of vasectomy in British men of this age and social group is between 5 and 10 percent, there seems to be a significantly higher proportion of men who have had this operation in the andropausal group. Not only are these patients on average five years younger than the rest, but often this operation appears to be the only risk factor present.

The most common time for the symptoms to appear is 10 to 15 years after the vasectomy. This time scale was confirmed independently by another group in London, who also showed a fall in testosterone levels at this time.[13] Other studies from Egypt and Belgium have shown that the amount of testosterone and one of its active fractions, dihydrotestosterone (DHT), in the semen, are reduced to one third by vasectomy.

Most of the studies of the effects of vasectomy on hormone production are relatively short term, taking place over three to five years at most.[14] Almost all were carried out 10 to 20 years ago, before vital factors such as sex hormone binding globulin (SHBG) and prostate specific antigen (PSA) were even being included in research studies. It's true they excluded any dramatic drop in total testosterone levels in the first five years after vasectomy, and some even showed an increase in DHT and follicle stimulating hormone (FSH).[15,16,17] However this indicates at least some hormonal changes occur even in this relatively short time scale, which could be taken to show some disturbance in testicular function, if not actual damage to its structure. Rather than vasectomy making you sexier, as suggested by one study recently, since DHT is not the primary hormone governing libido, a more likely explanation is that the pituitary gland is trying to compensate for impaired testosterone production by spurring the testis to greater activity, and increasing its turnover rate.

The surge in these two hormones could also explain why there have been several reports[18,19,20] of an increased number of cases of testicular cancer within the first four years after vasectomy, reaching a maximum after two, although there are other studies which contradict this.[21] This tumour increases at a rate of about 2 percent per annum, particularly in young men. It is more common when the testicles fail to descend, or they are damaged by mumps or trauma,[22] which is a condition also associated with raised FSHs. It has recently been linked to environmental estrogens, which, as already mentioned, may have a similar effect in contributing to testicular failure and high FSH levels.[23] It is fortunate that this is one form of cancer where great advances have been made in treatment.

Prostate cancer has also been linked to vasectomy in some studies but not in others.[24,25] Evidence is particularly conflicting here, but again, if it is proven, it could be explained by long-term hormonal disturbances. Reduced semen flow through the prostate has been suggested as another possible link, but seems unlikely, as vasectomy only reduces semen volume by 5 percent, and this form of cancer is not particularly common in men leading a celibate life, such as monks.

A typical andropausal man, for whom vasectomy seemed to be the most likely cause of his problems, is the 49-year-old doctor Alan:

I had a vasectomy 10 years ago. It was very painful and I had a lot of bruising. Suddenly, for no apparent reason, five years ago the bottom dropped out of my sex life. I used to be quite a flirt but then the sexual chemistry went and sex never entered my head, which was totally unlike me. About the same time, quite suddenly my morning erections disappeared and soon the evening ones went out of the door with them, especially when I wanted them most. This made me so worried that, a bit like my golf swing, which worsened at the same time, I got paralysis by analysis.

Also, while I used to really fizz all the time, I became a real slouch, stopped going to parties and started feeling old before my time. Then the circulation in my fingers and toes got quite bad even in the mild weather, and my feet started going numb. Even my joints started seizing up and got very stiff first thing in the morning and after golf or going running, both of which I used to enjoy, but they turned into a real bore and chore with all these symptoms.

At this stage I went and had a thorough checkup by my andrologist, who showed that the free testosterone in my blood was very much reduced. Capsules of testosterone by mouth gave a lot of improvement, but it wasn't until I started on the pellet implants into the buttock that the symptoms really went away and I got back to my old sexy self.

Best of all, my golf improved enormously. My handicap, which had deteriorated badly over the previous four years, went down by about five, and I started to beat the club champion and do well in away matches. The main difference was in my swing, which had become hasty and snatched, but on testosterone really flowed. Other people noticed the difference, especially my coach, and asked what I was on, but I haven't told them. I don't think it's my imagination either, because every five or six months when my implant is running down, my golf gets worse, as does my temper and sex life, and they are only restored by another shot of testosterone.

Especially when there are other causes of testicular failure, such as alcohol or mumps, vasectomy definitely seems to lower the age at which andropausal symptoms appear.

Vasectomy, the heart and circulatory disease

A great deal of work has been done on the possible link between vasectomy and heart and circulatory disease, and I find the evidence persuasive. It also coincides with my clinical experience and that of Dr Jens Møller and his successor Dr Michael Hansen.[26] It's true that a lot of the evidence implicating vasectomy in these conditions is from animal studies, but much of it is from experiments with monkeys, which are generally considered the closest one can get to the human condition.

Over 20 years ago it was shown that baboons given a high fat diet and inoculated with antibody producing proteins developed more arterial disease.[27] A few years after that the American queen of research in this field, Dr Nancy Alexander, and her colleague Dr Clarkson showed that diet-induced arterial disease developed more in vasectomized cynomolgus monkeys than in sham-operated controls. They therefore suggested, 'The immunological response to sperm antigens that often accompanies vasectomy may exacerbate atherosclerosis.' This is the form of arterial degeneration underlying most coronary heart disease.[28]

They followed up this early work with longer term studies which showed even more marked changes. This was largely confirmed in studies on primates by several other groups of researchers, particularly where the monkeys were overfed and underexercised, like the average Western male.

Although the link in monkeys between vasectomy and arterial disease is very clearly established, that in humans is much less so. Some studies, such as the Framingham study of heart disease risk factors in America, found an association with higher cholesterol levels, and one, on Korean men, higher heart attack rates.[29,30] Others, such as the Oxford Record Linkage study and a Kaiser Permanente study in California, did not.[21,31] The debate continues and the case has yet to be proved either way.

As well as the antibody related theories, there are a variety of reasons why vasectomy might contribute to circulatory problems. Anything which reduces the production of testosterone or antagonizes its actions is likely to contribute to these conditions. Dr Møller lists the reasons fully in his book *Testosterone Treatment of Circulatory Diseases*.[33] Mainly it is because of imbalance between the body's anabolic building up, restorative, energy producing activities and its catabolic, breaking down, energy consuming activities. As a result, the blood pressure and fat levels rise, blood clots happen more easily, flow of blood in the small blood vessel becomes sluggish, and the cells throughout the body become less efficient at taking up oxygen and using it. Consequently the natural rate of wear and tear on the heart and arteries escalates, and this leads to their premature aging.

The most dramatic case I saw where vasectomy seemed to be directly linked with circulatory problems was James, a young milkman from south London:

I was fine until I was 21 and then I got the mumps. It was so bad that my testicles swelled to the size of grapefruit, and I had to borrow a bra from my mom to carry them and ease the pain when I stood up. They seemed to settle down all right after an uncomfortable couple of weeks, but here must have been some damage because my wife had difficulty conceiving our first child and the clinic said my sperm count was low.

We made up for lost time, though, after that and had two more quickly, so I thought it was time to have a vasectomy. There was a little counseling beforehand, but no medical checks, as I looked and felt completely fit, and was only 34. No one asked me about the mumps, so I didn't think it could be relevant. The operation went fine and within a week I was back to my old sexy self, or even better.

Ten months later, though, I didn't feel nearly so good. I found that on my milk rounds, especially on cold winter mornings, I started getting really bad cramps in first my right calf and then my left. I was hobbling up the garden paths like an old man, and my rounds started taking longer and longer. I told my doctor about this and he said these symptoms sounded like not enough blood was getting to the leg muscles, but he had never seen this in anyone so young before.

The surgeon he sent me to was also very puzzled. He said surgery was needed, but I didn't fancy it and tried to treat myself by stopping smoking and exercising in a gym. This helped for a bit, but within a year I had to give in and have some of the furring up in the main artery in the right leg taken out.

This only helped for a couple of months and then I was back in the hospital having a whole series of complicated plumbing operations, trying to bypass the blockages with plastic tubes. None of these operations lasted more than a month or two and I couldn't do my rounds even when I was out of hospital because of the leg cramps. It got to the point of getting cramp in my right leg at night in bed and the surgeons started talking about amputation.

I was desperate and would rather have committed suicide than live life as a legless cripple. Still, I'm a philosophical sort of man who meditates and I still believed something would happen to save my legs. Well, I was lying in a bed on the surgical ward one morning going through The Sunday Times and there was this article about a Dr Møller in Copenhagen who was treating cases like mine with testosterone injections. Fate seemed to have been very kind to me, because a British doctor who was mentioned in the same article and seemed to believe in the treatment was working in the hospital just across the road from where I was.

He and my surgeon got together and agreed it was worth a try. After all, what had I got to lose, apart from my legs? Dr Carruthers really had to fight for the injections. Although my surgeon had given his permission, the hospital pharmacist said he thought the dose suggested was far too high and, among other dire warnings, that it might suppress my sperm production, which showed how little he knew about my case. This made the junior doctor who was told to give the injections, as no one else would, so nervous that he spilled half the dose out of the syringe each time.

Even so, it really was amazing. A few days after I started on the twice a week injections, my legs seemed to come alive again. The calf pain started taking longer and longer to come on, and I was able to leave the ward and take up my milk rounds, which badly needed my attention. One improvement I hadn't expected was that my erections returned nearly to normal after being very lame *affairs for a couple of years and I was only slightly tired for a couple of days after sex rather than being shattered for a week.*

There was a setback a couple of months later when the old plastic piping the surgeons had left in my right leg got infected and had to be taken out. This briefly made the blood flow in my right foot very bad indeed, so that gangrene nearly set in, but despite this, things went very well on the injections. My family doctor arranged for me to have them twice a week. I gave up going to the hospital, which seemed to lose interest in me when I didn't need any more surgery, and I wasn't sorry to stay out of their hands.

It's now over ten years since I started the testosterone treatment and I work out in a gym for an hour most days, swim twice a week, enjoy a great sex life and, having given up the stressful job of being a milkman, I am much happier teaching Tai Chi.

The funny thing is, though, none of the surgeons I used to consult seemed interested in why things went wrong so soon after the vasectomy or why I'm not in a wheelchair now, ten years after they said amputation was the only option left.

Most of the research studies on human vasectomy are unfortunately relatively short term, lasting only two to five years and ceasing before the complications I see 10 to 15 years later arise. One of the best conducted and reassuring studies was reported from Oxford in 1992. It found that:

> Vasectomy was not associated with an increased risk of testicular cancer or the other diseases studied. With respect to prostate cancer, while we found no cause for concern, longer periods of observation on large numbers of men are required.[34]

However this study did not cover impaired sexual function and other symptoms of andropause. Also, it is difficult when seeing case after case of severe menopausal and circulatory disease problems which appear to be directly associated with vasectomy, to be entirely convinced of its safety by the statistics of very artificial population studies.

Also, the vasectomized men are likely to be a very atypical self-selected group of clean living, well informed, health-conscious men in stable and loving relationships, who might be expected to enjoy better health all around, and yet are being compared with control populations who may lack these benefits.

Vested interests

There are powerful lobbies both inside and outside the medical profession with vested interests in maintaining the 'safe' image of vasectomy. First, doctors who have been promoting it for many years don't want to change their tune and to have to face the possibility of being in the wrong.

I saw this very clearly in 1979 when, alarmed by the similarities between Dr Moller's experience with his men and the evidence from the research in monkeys, I encouraged a very well informed and level-headed medical correspondent to write an article analyzing the vasectomy dilemma. Having done his homework very thoroughly, including a visit to Dr Møller's clinic in Copenhagen, he stated in his article: '*The view I have reached can be summarized as follows: with the present state of knowledge, I wouldn't dream of having a vasectomy myself.*' His conclusion was: 'It's safer to wait.'[4]

Although this article was cautious by journalistic standards, there was an immediate outcry by the medical establishment. The British Pregnancy Advisory Service dismissed the report as '*scare-mongering*' and other experts the journalist had consulted to get a balanced view before the publication asked him not to write about it at all.

I was involved in several radio and television debates on the question at the time, and the main argument of the antagonistic doctors was that vasectomy operations had been carried out for about a century and there had never been reports of an association between vasectomy and atherosclerosis in man. Would they have dismissed such evidence of arterial damage in monkeys, if it had been produced by a drug rather than an operation? It is more likely that there would have been a public outcry and the drug would have been taken off the market pending further research.

All this fierce opposition was before any questions were raised of one possibility of a link to testicular or prostatic cancer or to the hormonal disturbances involved in andropause. The steadfast support of the pro-vasectomy lobby was undeterred even by this possibility.

This reluctance of the medical profession to discuss vasectomy issues is likely to be even greater when the financial considerations of the vasectomy industry are taken into account.

In America, for example, it is estimated that over 500,000 vasectomies are carried out each year. Assuming that on average, with operative fees and all the associated costs such as testing for the absence of sperm three months after the operation, the cost of each vasectomy is $400, that is an annual turnover of $200 million. Add in another $15 million for the 1 percent of men who want the operation reversed at $3,000 dollars each, and a similar amount for treating the other short-term complications such as infection, pain, cysts, granulomas and so on, and this is quite a big business, well worth protecting.

There is, however, one consideration which might make American doctors think twice before continuing to recommend and perform vasectomies. If convincing evidence were produced that serious damage might result from either the antibody formation or hormonal changes which many studies have already shown to occur after the operation, it would open the floodgates for a torrent of highly emotive litigation cases. Even now, drug companies are caught up in defending some very large-scale group actions for everything from breast implants to drugs such as Thalidomide and Norplant.

In the brochure selling vasectomy in one large clinic in London the details are very brief, and so incomplete and inaccurate that they must surely flout advertising standards, let alone medical guidelines for informed consent to treatment. There are four brief paragraphs on possible hazards of the operation, which I quote in their entirety so that you can form your own impression on the fullness and fairness of this advice:

Complications, although very rare, can occur with any surgical procedure, however minor, and if you are worried about anything please feel free to call us for advice, or alternatively, if it is convenient, your own doctor.

There is no evidence of any long-term risk to men's health after vasectomy, in fact many couples find greater enjoyment once the risk of unwanted pregnancy has been removed. Orgasm and ejaculation are not affected.

Sperm continues to be produced by the testicles but its passage to the penis is blocked, so it is reabsorbed by the body, just as the body continually reabsorbs all unused cells.

semen no longer contains sperm.

Vasectomy has absolutely no effect on the production of male hormones, the
only difference is purely mechanical in that the semen no longer contains sperm.

Continuing with this limited 'purely mechanical' view, the form the
patient completes before the operation usually has more room for pay-
ment details than medical details.

Often immediately after signing this form, the man, who may be
only in his twenties or thirties, is led off, being given less time to
reconsider than he would have if he were buying a washing machine,
to have an operation with possible lifelong complications of which he
knows little, performed by a doctor of whom he knows less. Lawyers
defending such cases in the future may have a hard time proving that
the individual or organizations performing vasectomies under these
conditions were acting responsibly towards their patients.

It's not only doctors who don't want to hear any bad news about
vasectomy, though – governments also see it as the cheap and simple
answer to population control. This was seen in March 1991 in the
House of Lords, when Lord Anthony Blyth asked Her Majesty's
Government *whether they will take steps to discourage the vasectomy operation in view of the possible harmful effects in the long term.*

The Minister answering on behalf of the Government, Lord Henley,
immediately said:

No, my Lords. The decision as to whether or not a vasectomy should be
performed in any particular case is one for the patient and doctor concerned,
**taking full account of all the clinical issues involved. The patient is entitled
to have sufficient information on which to make a balanced judgement**. It is
for the doctor, as part of the counseling process, to decide what risks, **if any**,
the patient should be warned of and the terms in which any warning should be
given. (My emphasis.)

Under further questioning the Minister confirmed that the Government
was satisfied that men were being given adequate advice, discounted the
studies associating vasectomy with testicular or prostatic cancer and
omitted to mention any of the studies relating to circulatory disease.

Another Lord was of the opinion:

If there was any evidence of harmful effects from this comparatively minor operation, whether in the short or long term, should not the Chief Medical Officer of the Department [of Health] inform general practitioners of that fact? As he has not taken that step, am I entitled to assume that there are no such dangers?

The Minister confirmed he was.

I entirely agree with critics who say that the evidence against vasectomy is not conclusive yet and much more research is needed. However, as elsewhere in this book, I have deliberately made discussion of the topic provocative to stimulate research and informed debate. Particularly in relation to andropause, those who have had vasectomies should not be too alarmed, because symptoms generally respond very well to testosterone treatment. However, sometimes higher doses seem needed in this situation and, because the antibody changes are not reversible, treatment may need to be prolonged.

Also, reversing the vasectomy is not recommended, unless it is needed to restore fertility. This might even stir up a fresh storm of antibody production. It is also quite an expensive operation and there are only a few surgeons who have the expertise needed for this delicate form of microsurgery, which even in the most experienced hands has its own range of postoperative complications.

Vasectomy is a common operation and even if it results in short-term complications in a small number of people, or it has only a slight influence on the long-term chances of developing a serious illness such as prostate cancer,[35] this makes it important that we learn much more about it, and that people who have had it done, or are considering it, are better informed.[36]

In a recent TV documentary entitled 'If I were Prime Minister,' the feminist Germaine Greer said in her usual tongue-in-cheek, confrontational style that the first law she would enact would be to vasectomize all males on their eighteenth birthday. As she didn't wish to appear uncivilized, however, she would include a clause that for good behavior towards women over the following ten years, the men could apply to have their stored pre-vasectomy semen samples back.

Apart from what the men's movement would have to say on the subject, the feminists might well find that by the end of this probationary period, the resulting mass andropause might mean that most of the suitable mates had little interest in sex or procreation. Because the younger the age the vasectomy is performed, the greater the immune response, Germaine's suggestion is undesirable on every ground known to mankind: humanitarian, social, sexual and above all, medical.

The first recorded vasectomy was by a British surgeon, Sir Astley Cooper, who in 1823 vasectomized his dog.[37] My clinical experience over the past 15 years has made me firmly of the opinion that it shouldn't even happen to a dog. If you or a friend are thinking of having the knot of vasectomy tied, my earnest advice to you would be: Don't!

Having answered at least some of the questions about how male menopause or andropause happens, and the part which vasectomy may play, it's time to find out the good news: that it can usually be safely and effectively treated by giving testosterone.

Chapter six

Testosterone replacement therapy (TRT)

TRT is only one of a broad range of methods for preventing and treating andropause. Often, however, it proves the key to recovery and puts men in a more positive frame of mind to undertake the other necessary steps, such as managing stress, drinking less, losing weight and exercising.

Before deciding whether TRT is suitable and what additional treatments are needed to maximize its effects, the physician prescribing it will need to undertake a detailed 'work up.' When you go to him, your health history should be taken carefully and fully first. You must discuss factors which might have damaged the testes or stopped them functioning properly, such as non-descent, inflammations or orchitis such as mumps, vasectomy and other traumas, and local anatomical abnormalities.

Then there needs to be an 'Andropause Check List' similar to the one given in the second chapter (see pages 49–50). This will establish whether you have the symptoms which could be attributed to andropause and how severe they are, as well as giving a baseline to measure the effects of treatment.

Next comes a lifestyle and stress assessment questionnaire, which assesses the health history and lifestyle factors such as alcohol intake, diet, exercise, relaxation, smoking habits and stress related factors.

After this comes a physical check, with special emphasis on the heart and arteries, testicles and penis, and a digital rectal examination of the prostate gland. For those over 50, it is advisable to have a transrectal ultrasound examination of the prostate in addition to the mandatory prostate specific antigen (PSA) blood test which is the best overall early warning system for prostate cancer and an essential screening test before considering treatment with testosterone. The ultrasound examination is, however, quite expensive and seldom popular and newer advances in PSA testing measuring total and free forms of PSA may make it necessary less often.

The case for early detection of prostate cancer is still being fiercely debated. In my first 1,000 patients, six cases of early noninvasive prostate cancer were found prior to testosterone treatment and only three developed it during treatment, when it was picked up by the six-monthly screen at an early, treatable stage. In both cases this is a lower incidence than would be expected in a group of men with the majority over 50 years old, and would suggest that, by providing the benefit of this screening, testosterone treatment is overall more likely to save lives from prostate cancer than to cause it.

Finally, a detailed fasting morning blood profile, including a hormone profile, full biochemistry with checks on the liver, kidneys, blood fats and sugar, and hematological measurements of the red and white cells, is carried out in the laboratory. The hormone measurements include the total testosterone and the SHBG, the protein in the blood which limits its action, from which the active fraction, the Free Androgen Index (FAI), can be calculated by dividing the first by the second and multiplying by 100 to give a percentage. This key factor should normally be in the range of 70 to 100 percent, and andropausal symptoms are almost always present when it falls below 50 percent.

For reasons already mentioned (see pages 67–8), while the total testosterone level is often normal, even if in the lower part of the range, the FAI is usually significantly reduced before treatment and is the most reliable hormonal marker of andropause. Without it, no assessment of a man with symptoms which might be related to andropause is complete.

Also measured in the hormone profile are the two pituitary gland hormones which stimulate the testes, the follicle stimulating hormone (FSH) and luteinizing hormone (LH). For the reasons described previously (see page 63), the former, against textbook theory, is usually raised more than the latter in many, but not all, cases of andropause.[2]

Another important hormone which should be included in the initial screening is one from the pituitary gland, prolactin, which stimulates breast milk production in women. It also acts as a natural contraceptive, reducing fertility while women are breastfeeding and helping to space out pregnancies. It may be raised in both sexes during periods of stress, which reduces fertility and can lower testosterone production in the male.

Very occasionally, there is a benign tumor of the pituitary called a prolactinoma, which produces large amounts of this hormone, and testosterone levels fall dramatically. This results in loss of libido and potency, and all the other signs of testosterone deficiency. One positive benefit of the detailed hormonal profiling carried out in all cases before starting testosterone treatment is that these tumors are detected at an early stage, therefore other side effects of the pituitary enlargement, such as headaches and impaired vision due to pressure on the optic nerves, are left. Fortunately, in the five cases seen in my first 1,000 patients, their symptoms were dramatically relieved by an antiprolactin drug called bromocriptin, which also shrank the enlarged pituitary gland back to normal size and avoided neurosurgery.

One of the estrogen group of hormones, estradiol (E2), is also included in the blood test and sometimes gives interesting information. Since it is produced in men mainly by the metabolism of testosterone, where that is in short supply it often goes down. When the patient is overweight, there is a tendency for more of the natural testosterone, and even testosterone given as treatment, to be converted to E2; this may then rise to a level where it causes breast enlargement and may also reduce the action of the parent hormone. This paradoxical reaction only seems to happen in a few patients. It can be reduced by a variety of changes in the treatment given, as some forms of testosterone are not converted to E2. There is also scope for investigating the use of the newer forms of anti-estrogen drugs, which are proving very effective in the treatment of breast cancer in women and show promise as an additional weapon in the treatment of andropausal men.[3,4]

Unfortunately, as yet there is no convenient blood test for the estrogen mimics, xeno-estrogens, or the anti-androgens already discussed, which may be playing a part in bringing on andropause. Such a test would be a great boon to mankind, both in relation to this condition and falling sperm counts.[5]

When the results of all these tests are in, which can be done within a day in some clinics, a second session is needed with your doctor.

At this you go over the results together and draw up an overall treatment program. This is usually not just getting testosterone, but also involves active input on your part, modifying your lifestyle in a variety of ways, reducing weight and alcohol intake, changing to boxer shorts and adopting strategies to cope with stress, if necessary.

Always remember, *you* are in the pilot's seat and in overall control of your life. In relation to testosterone treatment, after having the risks and likely benefits explained and your questions clearly answered, you have to decide whether to have the treatment, and literally call the shots.

TRT can be given in the form of injections, pills and pellets, and through the skin as creams and patches. The decision of whom to treat, with which preparation, in what doses and for how long, must rest with the individual physician, as part of a joint and informed venture with the patient. Here I can only give my personal experience, my views derived from it and a review of the extensive literature on the subject.

When asked where the testosterone comes from, doctors sometimes tell patients that it is extracted from Peruvian bulls' testicles in the mating season, both to explain the cost of the treatment and maximize the placebo effect, but that's a lot of bull, really. Testosterone is made synthetically from cholesterol, the same raw material as the body uses to produce it. The current cost of these preparations is usually roughly two to three times that of equivalent estrogen preparations used for female HRT, but hopefully as TRT is used more often, drug companies will be able to reduce this sex hormone discrimination against men.

When testosterone was first produced back in 1935, doctors realized that it was poorly absorbed and rapidly broken down in the liver, so it would not be effective when taken by mouth. So it was necessary to both bypass the liver and to chemically modify the molecule to slow its rate of absorption and breakdown. One of the most effective ways was to attach side chains to the testosterone molecule and form compounds called esters. The longer the side chain in general, the slower the rate of breakdown.[6] But how to administer it?

Injections

Injections of pure testosterone were tried early on, but were found to work for only two hours. Although the effects were good while they lasted, some means had to be found of getting a longer period of action if the treatment was to become popular.

The first attempt at this was by making an ester called testosterone propionate. Having a short side chain, it only lasted two or three days, but this enabled it to be used clinically, even if it meant injections two or three times a week. This was the preparation used in 1944 by Heller and Myers (see pages 18–19) to demonstrate for once, if not for all, that male menopause is due to testosterone deficiency. They also showed, in a controlled trial using placebo injections of sesame oil, how the symptoms of this very real hormonal disorder, including erection problems, could be abolished by TRT.[7]

After the Second World War, research on finding newer and more effective medications got under way. An ester called testosterone enanthate (Primo-Teston Depot) was produced by the Schering company in Berlin and found to be clinically very effective. Having a longer side chain, it was broken down even more slowly and injections lasted two or three weeks.

It was this medication which Dr Jens Møller used with such impressive results in his clinic in Copenhagen for over 30 years in treating circulatory disorders.[8] It was given in high doses of 250 mg every two weeks or even once a week in severe cases. As in the case of James (see pages 90–2), it usually gives a dramatic relief of symptoms within a few days.

It is presently the best injectable form widely available in the United States and has produced excellent results in a 'Hormonal Healthcare Center' I established and was medical director of in Hawaii. The patients I saw there showed just the same symptoms as the ones coming for treatment to London – it seems that andropause can strike with equal force even in the 'Paradise Islands.'

There are other esters available, and cocktail mixtures of esters such as the commonly used Sustenon, but they seem to have no advantage over testosterone enanthate. They all share the problem of giving a peak of testosterone after a few hours which is higher than needed and might have some harmful effects, for example on the liver.

The surplus can also be converted to estrogen, which is again undesirable. The level then falls steadily over two or three weeks to a low point which may be insufficient to relieve andropausal or circulatory symptoms. The patient is aware of these ups and downs of the testosterone levels, and his life can be a rollercoaster ride of emotional and sexual highs and lows. Also the injections, usually given into the buttock, are somewhat painful and quite expensive, which limit their availability and popularity, especially for long-term use.

To overcome some of these disadvantages, several very promising new injections are now undergoing clinical trials. They offer the possibility of an extended action lasting between two and four months per shot. This would also get around the problems of poor absorption of the oral forms, where 50 to 80 percent of this expensive hormone goes down the toilet, the problem of fluctuating blood levels and the natural dislike of most men to taking medicine two to three times a day, perhaps for years on end.

Pills

It was a tragedy for testosterone treatment that the first oral form to be produced back in 1935 was methyl testosterone. As I've already explained, it was effective but had some very dangerous side effects which have tarnished the medical image of testosterone to this day. Even though we now have much safer medications, this one can be obtained over the counter, without prescription, in many parts of the Far East and is still the only oral form of testosterone available in the United States. Why is that watchdog of American medicine, the Federal Drug Administration (FDA), still asleep in allowing this drug onto the market, while keeping the much better and safer varieties of this vital hormone out?

The harmful side effects of methyl testosterone include damage to the liver cells, resulting in cysts and even cancer. Unlike other forms of testosterone, it also sends up blood fat levels, particularly cholesterol. This is why one of the doctors who is a leading authority on testosterone, Professor Eberhard Nieschlag from Munich, firmly stated in his 1990 review of different forms of testosterone treatment:

Because of the side effects methyl testosterone should no longer be used therapeutically, in particular since effective alternatives are available. The German Endocrine Society declared methyl testosterone obsolete in 1981 and the German Federal Health Authority ruled that methyl testosterone should be withdrawn from the market in 1988. In other countries, however, methyl testosterone is still in use, a practice which should be terminated.[9]

These are strong words indeed, but ones with which I entirely agree.

The dangers of this compound being foisted on a largely unsuspecting public were vividly brought home to me recently by the story of an engineer called Ken who had been forced to go overseas to get his testosterone supplies:

At the tender age of 37 I started to feel a severe lack of energy and lost interest in everything. Life just seemed too much bother. My work as a service engineer involved new techniques using computers and I started only just being able to keep up with the rapidly advancing technology, instead of being ahead of it as I had been before. This and my reduced libido and increasing difficulty with erections all combined to make me feel mildly depressed and generally flat. Even my physique started to deteriorate, and playing squash, or even carrying a heavy toolbox up stairs, began to make me puff and pant.

After trying all sorts of things from hypnosis to acupuncture and herbal remedies for three years, I went to my family doctor, who checked me over. After a blood test he said my testosterone was below normal, but said he didn't advise any treatment. When I persisted, he got quite irritable and said, 'Well, your work takes you around the world a lot – why don't you get some on your travels?'

At the time I was spending alternate months in Thailand, so on my very next trip I went into a drug store over there, where you can get about anything over the counter with no questions asked, and got some 'Metesto.' The label on the bottle said that each white tablet contained 25 mg of Methyltestosterone, made in Bangkok, so it sounded like just what I needed. The instructions were in Thai, so as there were 100 tablets in the bottle and I wanted them to last a month, I decided that one three times a day would be the right dose and away I went.

I must say, within a few days I began to feel much better, quite my old self. My wife said I looked better when I got home at the end of the month, but the job in Thailand ended and when the pills ran out, all the old symptoms came back.

This time I went to a specialist in the field, who after detailed tests said my testosterone was now only a tenth of what it should be, and the form of testosterone I'd taken had caused some hopefully temporary liver damage and raised my blood cholesterol. He put me on a safer medication also taken by mouth and within three months I was feeling fine again, and my liver function and cholesterol were back down to normal.

Now, six years later, I'm having pellet implants of testosterone, which keep me feeling very well and fit. The funny thing is that my wife, who is going through menopause and couldn't keep up with my libido, which has returned to what it was before my problems started, is having just a touch of testosterone in with her estrogen pellet implants, so that we have ended up on the same medicine.

There are two much safer oral medications available in Britain and the rest of Europe, South Africa and Australia, and I have used them both extensively over the past seven years in treating patients with symptoms of andropause.

The stronger of the two medications is a long chain fatty acid ester called testosterone undecanoate, first used clinically in the mid 1970s. It is known under the trade names given to it by the Belgian company Organon which makes it: Restandol in Europe and Andriol in the rest of the world, including Canada where it has only recently come onto the market. It is made in small reddish-brown oval capsules containing 40 mg of the ester, equivalent to 25 mg of testosterone. It is dissolved in arachis oil so that when taken after a meal it is absorbed by the fat droplets coming from the small intestine, goes into the lymphatic drainage and bypasses the liver so that it is not immediately broken down. Peak serum levels are reached after two to four hours and most is broken down by eight hours, so that this form needs to be taken two or, ideally, three times a day.

The other safe oral medication is mesterolone (Proviron), which comes in the form of white 25 mg pills made by the German firm Schering. Unlike testosterone itself and other testosterone derivatives, which are broken down to both an active product called dihydrotestosterone (DHT) and estrogens, mesterolone only produces raised levels of the former, which makes it a weaker androgen, particularly in relation to improving both libido and potency. However, for unknown reasons, it still sometimes seems to work when the undecanoate fails so it is a useful reserve form, especially when a patient wishes to maintain or even improve fertility, which the other preparations may temporarily suppress. It can, for instance, help young men with the *'locker room syndrome'* described in Chapter Eight to feel more 'macho.' An example of this kind of case is Nick:

Although I'm 22 now, I managed to finish my course at university, where all my friends claimed to have scored one or more times with girls, without me quite managing it. Since someone said my penis seemed rather small in the showers one day after a rugby match two years ago, it really seems to be shrinking. This shattered my confidence and I stopped getting firm erections even when I masturbated.

I felt so bad about this that I gave up athletics and football, and became what you call a computer nerd, preferring the Internet to basketball. Although I took some drugs in my teens, I think it was more a very bad attack of glandular fever I had when I was 15 that caused the trouble. Because I was very worried about this I went to see a psychiatrist who tried some tranquilizers on me which didn't seem to help at all and probably made the erection problems worse. Then I saw a urologist, who took one look at me and said it was a perfectly normal size and I should forget about it.

As I couldn't, I went to see an andrologist who took a careful history, examined me fully and did a detailed hormone profile. This showed a slight decrease in the free, active testosterone, perhaps due to the glandular fever or the stress of my final university exams, and he said that he would give me a short course of a mild form of testosterone called Proviron to boost my confidence.

That was six months ago, and it seemed to give me a kick start and make me feel confident enough to start a relationship with a girl, with whom I'm having regular sex. She really is very complimentary about my penis and it seems to respond very well to this; even though I've been off the Proviron for three months now.

Pellets

Pellets made of crystals of pure testosterone fused together under pressure or by heat have been made by the Belgian company Organon and used clinically since 1937. The safety and effectiveness of this preparation can be judged from the fact that it has been used virtually unchanged for nearly 60 years and has an excellent track record. Under a local anesthetic, six to ten of the small cylindrical pellets, each containing 200 mg of testosterone, are introduced through a single large needle deep into the fat of the buttock. Aside from the initial sting of the local anesthetic, it is a painless procedure taking about half an hour. It gives good levels of testosterone for around six months, and is still the longest acting and most steadily effective form of TRT available.[10] It also gives the most sustained and natural pattern of testosterone related hormones, with no excessive rise in DHT. The only occasional side effect is that one or more of the pellets tracks to the surface and discharges itself, after which the puncture site heals over again.

Many patients enjoy the freedom from taking the testosterone undecanoate capsules on which they usually start and obtain very effective relief of andropausal symptoms from the pellet implant. This is not a placebo reaction because it not only goes on working year after year, but even when a patient does not know what to expect, he experiences a gradual return of symptoms every six months or so, which is obvious both to himself and his family. This is often reported as 'My battery is running down and I need a top up.'

The long-term safety of correctly applied testosterone treatment in general, and this method in particular, has been clearly demonstrated by over 1,000 implants performed in over 300 patients attending my clinic who have been kept free of andropausal symptoms by the implants for up to ten years now, including three who have been treated for primary testicular failure since their teens with testosterone implants for 30, 40 and 57 years respectively. Ben, the last, was one of the first patients in Britain to be treated by this method and his story is part of its history:

When I was a young boy, only 12 in fact, my father spotted that my testicles were not in the usual place, having stayed up in my abdomen. This was very worrying to me and my parents who thought I was never destined to go through puberty or become a proper man because I was suffering the then untreatable condition of what was called 'primary hypogonadism.'

Then at the age of 17, with no sign of a breaking voice or body hair like the other boys in my class at school, I had a lucky break by being referred to a Dr Peter Bishop, who was Professor of Endocrinology at Guy's Hospital in London. He had just been over to the USA and learned of a technique of implanting pellets of pure crystalline testosterone which they were using over there.

From 1944 onward I started having the implants every six months into the side of my thighs, which was where they did them then. I got to know the clinic staff very well over the years, and they shared my pleasure in going through a normal, though somewhat late puberty, getting a job in the civil service, and then getting married at the age of 24. I had a happy sexually active married life, but with no children, of course, as the undescended testicles never worked and had to be removed when I was 26 to prevent them developing cancer.

At the end of every six months, I could feel the effects of the testosterone beginning to wear off. At about the same time I started to feel tired, my interest in making love to my wife would die away and it became too much like hard work. The most severe of these withdrawal symptoms, though, were violent headaches, like bad migraine. Also my penis seemed to shrink in and my confidence just went. Within a fortnight of each implant I felt like a young lad again and generally more 'cocksure' in every sense of the term. Girls looked nicer, my beard growth speeded up, my blood felt hotter and I seemed to glow with health.

Imagine my surprise and distress then when after being on the implants for over 47 years, I got a letter from the doctor who had taken over running the clinic to say that because of 'extreme cash pressures' they would no longer be providing an implant service and we would have to go to our family doctors to get injections every two or three weeks. Sometimes when I'd missed an appointment at the clinic, I'd had to try these injections for a month or two and, like the couple of hundred other regulars at the clinic, I knew they were not nearly as good or as convenient and certainly didn't give anything like the same steady reliable benefits as the implants. It seemed a rather cynical move on some administrator's part to shift the expense of our testosterone treatment off the hospital budget onto that of family doctors around the country.

Then I had my second lucky break and found a private doctor who was using the good old-fashioned pellet system. Everything is fine again now. I've been having the implants for another ten years, taking me over the half century mark. This must say something about the safety of testosterone treatment as my six monthly blood checks show my body chemistry is fine, especially the prostate test, which is as low as that of a 30-year-old.

Although I've retired now, I feel very fit and have taken up growing moustaches of different styles, which I think make me look rather distinguished really. Certainly my wife must be very tickled by them, as we had sex five times last week, which is not bad for an over 70-year-old who got off to a slow start in this area of his life.

Patches

Different nationalities seem to have different preferred methods of taking medicines. The British persevere with their oral tradition and have a pill for every ill. The Americans are more impatient and direct, preferring injections, and have a shot for every spot. The French are a more sensuous race, favoring suppositories and creams; they find a pessary very necessary and that a balm can make you calm. So it was naturally a French doctor, Dr Jayle, who as long ago as 1942 prepared a cream containing testosterone and it became quite popular, with Frenchmen at least, who claimed it did wonders for their *amour propre*.[11] Frenchwomen were not so enamored with this treatment because they found that the cream rubbed off onto them and while it enhanced desire, it put hair on their thighs and face, as reported by another French doctor, Dr Delanoe, in 1984.[12]

Undeterred, the French went on to develop a gel called Andractim, containing dihydrotestosterone (DHT), which, they assured the ladies, was quite safe because it was rapidly absorbed even when rubbed over a large area of manly chest twice a day. To make doubly sure, however, they recommended controlling passion for 10 minutes after application of the gel and then having a shower to wash off any excess. We must just hope they read and obey the writing on the tube every time, because men usually need a large dose of testosterone to improve andropausal symptoms, while in women a little goes a long way! Also DHT alone, while promoting facial and body hair growth, as seen with mesterolone treatment, which trebles DHT levels, has generally less effect on libido or erection problems in most cases than the pellet implant, which leaves DHT levels unchanged.

Recently, a new cream containing pure testosterone, called Androgel, has been released in the USA, and appears to be one of the best transdermal preparations yet produced. Rumor has it that Wall Street traders are slapping some on each other's backs before they go into crucial sales meetings, and swear by the boost it gives their competitive edge. However, this is still a very expensive preparation, and has not been released in the rest of the world yet, so it is difficult to judge its long-term effectiveness.

The big breakthrough in patches came with the development by an American, Dr Virgil Place, working for the ALZA Corporation in Palo

Alto, California. He developed a whole series of transdermal therapeutic systems (TTS), including the HRT patch for women, called
Estraderm. As he told me once, he had 'a heck of a job' getting the
female patch accepted. It was rather like the incredulity that Sir Walter
Raleigh met with when he returned from America with a new drug
delivery system consisting of the leaves of a plant which you dried,
rolled up and then set fire to before you inhaled the smoke. However,
like that system, once the HRT patch was marketed properly, it soon
became a multimillion pound industry world-wide. Unlike smoking,
though, it is a healthy habit giving benefit to millions of menopausal
women.

As Dr Place explained, however, developing the male patch and getting it accepted gave even greater problems.[13] First, a much larger dose
of testosterone has to be delivered in the hormone-deficient male than
the minute amount of estrogen needed in the menopausal female.
Second, the only area of skin thin enough for the testosterone to get
through was thought to be the scrotum, and there the skin was hairy
and so sensitive that you couldn't use adhesives, which are an irritant,
to stick them on with. So he came up with a patch called Testoderm,
which was applied in the morning to the shaved scrotum, itself a tick-
lish business, and was repeated each day. This appliance of science
became known as the 'Bals-Pratsch Patch,' named after Dr. Monika
Bals-Pratsch of Munich University, who in 1986 was the first to report
a clinically successful trial using the system.[14]

However, extensive trials of the system showed that it was inconvenient to use, likely to be expensive long term and had the theoretical disadvantage of producing an abnormal hormone profile. This was
because the scrotal skin also happens to be the only area of the body
rich in an enzyme called 5-alpha reductase, which converted the
testosterone to DHT while it was being absorbed. For all these reasons, Testoderm was never marketed on a commercial basis and has
now been superseded by patches with an even more efficient delivery
system which can be applied to any area of skin, even, like the female
HRT patch, to the buttock.

Antroderm, as the new patch is called, was developed by an
American company called Theratech Inc., and was marketed world-
wide by SmithKline Beecham.[15] It is a very promising development and
has undergone multi-center controlled clinical trials showing its

safety and efficacy in studies at Johns Hopkins University, and University of Utah and Karolinska Hospital in Stockholm, Sweden. It was found that two patches applied every night for periods of up to a year restored a normal hormonal pattern to nearly 100 'hypogonadal' men aged 15 to 65. The main side effects were limited to slight skin irritation at the site of the patches, a common complication of the female HRT patch. With this excellent research data behind it, the patches received Federal Drug Administration marketing approval in America with a speed that surprised even the manufacturers. Several other skin and scrotal patches have been released, the latest being 'Andropatch' (Testoderm), marketed by Ferring Pharmaceuticals, causing renewed media interest in the whole subject of andropause.

Here again controversy arises, because to meet with orthodox medical approval the manufacturers have obtained a license to market the new patches for the treatment of male 'hypogonadism,' which is a flexible term meaning different things to different doctors. They might well take the view quoted in Lewis Carroll's *Through the Looking Glass*: '"When I use a word," Humpty Dumpty said in a rather scornful tone, "it means just what I choose it to mean – neither more nor less."'

The conventional medical definition of hypogonadism would be where the total plasma testosterone is below the 'normal range.' But we have seen, and the majority of andrologists would agree, that it is the free, biologically active testosterone, as represented by the FAI, which in fact determines the adequacy of testosterone for the body's needs. Strict application of the former definition, as my research has shown, would exclude over 85 percent of patients with clear-cut andropausal symptoms from the benefits of treatment with any testosterone medication, including the patch.

Also, there is no real agreement about what the so-called normal range actually is, particularly in men over the age of 40. Professor Alex Vermeulen from the University of Ghent in Belgium has spent a large part of his long and distinguished career trying to establish this very point.[16] He has found that studies to establish plasma levels of the male hormones at different ages can get totally different results according to whether or not you include or exclude either sick or exceptionally healthy men, particularly those over the age of 60. This does not include the effects on the levels of tissue testosterone and DHT, which are more than halved. How do you establish a normal range to diagnose a condition, when 50, 60 or 70 percent or more may be suffering some related symptoms which could be helped by treatment?

Add to that the variation of testosterone levels as measured in the same sample in different laboratories using a wide variety of methods, often giving different results, and the textbook definition of 'hypogonadism' loses most of its meaning in the real clinical world. The situation is made even worse by the fact that the units in which all the sex hormones are measured differ between America and Europe, two great nations divided by uncommon units, so that frequently doctors on one side of the Atlantic don't know what reference ranges the other side are using.

Finally, we don't know how age changes the concentrations needed in different body tissues for the many and varied actions of testosterone and its derivatives. This is especially so in 'High-T' males, who only feel and function well on high levels of the hormone. These may need to be as high, if not higher than that seen in young fit men, rather than the amount found in the men over 40 who usually develop the symptoms. Like racing cars, they need to run on high octane fuel from the start to the finish of life's race.

The idea is emerging that we should give the patients the benefit of the doubt, and rather than relying on laboratory tests alone, try to relieve the characteristic andropausal symptoms with a therapeutic trial of testosterone. This needs to be done over a three-month period at least, and not with just a single shot of testosterone as has been tried in some university clinics. The body and mind need time to recover from the multiple long-term problems which testosterone deficiency can cause.

Results of TRT

The results of the study carried out on the first 1,000 of now over 2,000 of my andropausal patients in London gives, I think, good evidence that andropause is a reality, due to either an absolute or relative deficiency of testosterone, which can be treated safely and effectively with TRT.

The age of the subjects ranged from 31 to 80, the mean being 54, which indicates the diverse range of often overlapping factors which can bring on andropause. This gives it a wider age span than the traditional 45-55 which covers the onset of menopause in women. Since the symptoms had on average been present for around four years, however, the peak time of onset is identical.

The mental symptoms included fatigue in 76 percent, depression in 60 percent and increased irritability in 54 percent. The physical symptoms were aches, pains and stiffness, particularly in the hands and feet, in over 55 percent, night sweats in 50 percent and dryness and thinning of the skin in 39 percent. Sexual problems were present in over 90 percent, and included loss of both libido and erectile problems in around 80 percent.

In addition to the changes associated with aging, possible overlapping causes of these symptoms were stress in 60 percent; alcohol in 35 percent; a wide variety of medicines known to affect potency or which might lower testosterone in over 30 percent; operations or injuries which might damage the testes or impair erection, especially in the 20 percent with vasectomy, another 30 percent; infections such as mumps, smoking and obesity all at around 20 percent each.

This study, which was passed by the local ethics committee, took the form of a cross-sectional survey of the initial profile of this group of andropausal men, and then a retrospective audit of the results obtained by treating the patients initially with either oral testosterone undecanoate (TU – Restandol) or mesterolone (ME – Pro-Viron). It was found most effective to give the main dose of either oral treatment before breakfast, and a second dose with lunch. Both groups also received advice on general measures such as relaxation, drinking less, weight loss, exercise and wearing loose-fitting boxer shorts, and were followed up with the same range of detailed blood tests, full hormonal profiles, prostate specific antigens, blood pressure, weight and andropause symptom checklist.

Depending on response and the patients' wishes, after three to six months of either of the oral treatments, testosterone pellet implantation (TI) was offered as a choice for long-term treatment.

Clinically, there was an overall feeling of increased vitality and well-being in all groups. Drive and assertiveness were observed to be increased by both the patients and their partners, but not to the point of aggression. In fact many became happier, less irritable and generally easier to live with, and felt they were coping better at work and in their family lives.

Increased hair growth, particularly on the chest and pubic region, was often noted by the patients. There was no hair loss from the scalp, and many felt the condition of their hair and skin had improved, with a markedly enhanced ability to tan. A few noted their hair color had been restored. Penile enlargement and increased genital sensitivity were also noted with satisfaction by some.

Unpleasant side effects were minimal, and limited to mild gastric irritation in a few patients on TU and the occasional loss of one or more pellets when the implants were rejected, which is an infrequent complication of this otherwise very convenient and effective form of treatment.

Andropausal symptom scores all fell significantly statistically and total sexual activity, which includes both intercourse and masturbation, increased in all three treatment groups. The benefits were most marked in the implant group, particularly in terms of increasing sexual activity and improving the relationship with the partner. Depression measures also decreased and went from being moderately severe back into the normal range.

On the safety side, blood pressures were unchanged or even fell slightly in the TU group after six months' treatment. There were no adverse changes in blood fat patterns, glucose, liver function tests or any part of the detailed blood profile. In particular, the early warning sign for prostate cancer, the prostate specific antigen (PSA), did not rise above the normal range at repeated tests up to ten years, there were no signs of enlargement of the prostate clinically or on ultrasound scanning. The three cases of prostate cancer which developed were picked up at an early, easily treatable stage.

Although a degree of placebo effect cannot be excluded in this type of study, it would not seem to account for either the magnitude or duration of the benefits, or the hormone changes in the expected direction which accompanied them. The very low test doses of either of the two oral testosterone derivatives given for the first month were effectively a form of placebo treatment. The subjects usually failed to respond to this, yet the placebo effect should then have been strongest. Only when the dose was doubled or trebled to therapeutic levels did they begin to feel the benefits.

Also with the implant treatment, it was only after two weeks, when the testosterone levels had risen, that the effects were experienced.

Similarly, the observed benefits wore off and the symptoms, especially of fatigue, returned at about six months after the implant, when the hormone levels were dropping back toward their pretreatment values.

Difficulties of double blind trials

George Bernard Shaw once remarked that doctors pour medicines, of which they know little, into patients, of whom they know less. In clinical practice today, the situation is probably much the same, but knowledge of the former is increasing, often at the expense of the latter.

Medicine has now become much more of a science than an art. What once seemed simple is now complex. Doctors used to give medicines and observe carefully what happened. If the patients seemed to improve, they continued to use the treatment and if they didn't, they stopped. Hormone treatments such as cortisone, thyroid hormone and insulin were introduced in this way because the benefits were blindingly obvious to doctors and patients alike, and could make the difference between life and death. In his use of testosterone in patients with severe arterial disease in the legs, Dr Jens Møller saw the dramatic benefits of treatment in preventing amputation for gangrene in the same light as giving insulin to diabetics, and felt it would be unethical not to do so.

However, medical science, before it will accept any line of treatment as being proven, now demands what are known as 'double blind control trials.' This means that the treatment on trial has to be given without either the patient or the doctor knowing whether active or placebo drug is being given at any one time. Depending on the design of the study, whether it is cross-sectional, longitudinal, crossover or the exotic 'Latin-square,' this can double, or even quadruple, the number of patients, the time needed and often the cost as well. It obviously limits the number of doctors who, without extensive and expensive research facilities, are able to undertake such studies, record and analyze them in the required statistical detail, and makes them more susceptible to commercial pressures in the design and interpretation of their studies.

Also, you now need to tell the patients that they are taking part in a trial and for them to give informed consent. This makes them dubious about the medicine and in private practice patients want to be sure that the specialist they see is not acting 'blindly,' but giving them the best medicine for their particular case and that they are getting it right away. Where the medicine is effective in relieving their symptoms, in a double blind trial the patients usually know before the doctor does whether they are on the active drug or placebo. There is also the confounding effect of the other range of lifestyle modifications which the doctor will recommend in some patients and not in others and the variable placebo power of different doctors in encouraging the patients to undertake them.

The situation is even more difficult with testosterone treatment because, as was explained to me when I tried initially to get research funds, many of the medications have been around for between 20 and 50 years, so that they are not only out of patent protection, but in the case of pellet implants, out of the product license period. This limited the interest of drug companies in such products, unless there is a new and difficult-to-reproduce drug delivery system involved and they can see a large and guaranteed market.

Having said all this, some of the newer testosterone medications such as the long-acting injections and patches may prove to be sufficiently 'sexy' for the drug companies or medical research organizations to subsidize scientifically 'pure' trials. In the meantime we will probably have to present the relatively 'impure' evidence of the practical experience of patients on treatment, combined with evidence from the literature and the cross-sectional research information on changes in symptoms and hormone levels such as that reported in this chapter.

The data is there, carefully gathered over more than ten years in computerized format, testifying particularly to the safety and effectiveness of long-term testosterone treatment, and I cordially invite my medical colleagues from an academic medical background to examine, analyze and report on what I regard as a mine of interesting, important and exciting information.

A detailed analysis of this study, the lessons learned from it and how it fits in with the rapidly escalating amount of research data from all over the world supporting the theory and practice of testosterone treatment, is being published by Parthenon Books in the USA and UK under the title of 'ADAM – Androgen Deficiency in the Adult Male: Causes, diagnosis and treatment.'[17]

Safety factors

Concerns about the safety of the treatment naturally focus mainly on the prostate gland, the liver and the heart. In all these areas, except where methyl testosterone was used, long-term clinical experience in the 50 year in which a variety of testosterone treatments have been available, together with detailed reviews of the literature and the results of the serial investigations in this study, have been reassuring (see Chapter 11).

Some of the resistance to TRT which has arisen in the last two generations of physicians is undoubtedly due to the abuse of anabolic steroids by athletes and body-builders highlighted in a recent report. The occasional reports of mental and physical harm done by dangerous cocktails of these drugs being 'cycled' and 'stacked' in grossly excessive doses should not be allowed to detract from the excellent clinical experience over many years with carefully monitored therapeutic use. As the amounts taken by abusers are often 10 to 20 times the therapeutic doses, these illicit and thoroughly undesirable experiments appear to have proved that most anabolic steroids have a considerable margin of safety, for men at least.[18]

Also one could point to the use in multicenter WHO trials of high dose testosterone by injection as a male contraceptive. These injections in young healthy men to suppress sperm production give two or three times the natural hormonal level which is the target for older men with severe andropausal symptoms, and so provide a resounding vote of safety for testosterone treatment.[19]

The debate on whether testosterone treatment might initiate cancer of the prostate is closely comparable to the controversy about whether female estrogen replacement therapy would cause breast cancer. Just as most recent studies of HRT have shown little if any increase after up to 10 years' treatment with estrogens, 50 years' of treatment of hypogonadal patients with testosterone implants and 30 years of treatment with injections of testosterone enanthate do not show any rising incidence of prostate cancer of even benign hypertrophy.

Forty years ago, studies were reported of 200 men over the age of 45, 100 of whom received intensive androgen therapy with no increase in the incidence of prostatic cancer or benign hyperplasia.[20] A recent review article on androgens and carcinoma of the prostate summarized the present informed view by stating: '*It is extremely unlikely that androgens play a role in the initiation of prostate cancer.*'[21]

Also, the area to be screened in the case of the prostate is the size of the thumb and ultrasound pictures give a very clear view of wherever cancer might arise. By contrast, the breasts are much more difficult to screen, X-rays which may themselves be harmful have to be used and there is no sensitive blood test like the PSA which can be used to exclude breast cancer.

A generation ago, women were arguing the same case in relation to whether treatment of their menopausal symptoms was flying in the face of nature. Fortunately, against stiff medical opposition, based largely on groundless worries over safety, they won that fight.[22] Moreover, as already noted, as the many benefits of long-term estrogen treatment became apparent, largely through research work by clinician-based organizations such as the British Menopause Society, the interesting paradox arose that many alleged contraindications such as cardiovascular disease, became positive indications.

In summary it can be concluded that HRT for men is as safe, if not safer, than HRT for women. At least the men who have had the type of detailed 'well man' screen which is carried out prior to testosterone treatment know they are not harboring prostate cancer, while many of their friends of the same age may be hosts to this silent assassin without knowing it until it is too late.

Future directions in testosterone treatment

It seems certain that with the advent of the Testosterone Revolution, this is a hormone whose time has finally come, and that TRT for men will take its rightful and very necessary place alongside HRT with estrogen for women, as an integral part of preventive medicine in the twenty-first century. It is equally certain that new testosterone medications will have to be introduced, as none of those presently available is ideal.

As an alternative to these treatments, it may be possible to stimulate the body's own natural production of testosterone, to slow its use and breakdown or lessen the factors antagonizing its action.

One of the most exciting developments in this field has been the use of a drug to reduce the sex hormone binding globulin (SHBG), which as described in chapter four, binds testosterone and limits the amount of free, bio-available testosterone in the body. Studies in my London clinic over the last six years have shown how very small doses of this drug, danazol (Danol), can halve the SHBG,[23] and reverse the increases in this key factor that are caused by age,[24] low protein diets[25] and myriad other factors.

Especially when combined with testosterone, the drug, which had previously mainly been used in women, can restore a more youthful pattern of hormone balance, and greatly increase the effectiveness of treatment of andropause. This 'freedom for testosterone' now makes it possible to treat patients with very high levels of this binding protein, who were previously 'black holes' for the hormone, and failed to respond to even large doses. In some patients, the testosterone already produced by the body can be liberated and activated by this drug alone, and gives a form of testosterone-free testosterone treatment – an interesting therapeutic paradox.

Chapter seven

Sexual satisfaction

Sexual dissatisfaction was overall the most common complaint in both my heterosexual and homosexual andropausal patients (92 percent), along with their partners (84 percent). While in no way wishing to suggest that sex is the be all and end all of a marriage or other long-term partnership, as one patient put it, 'It is more than just the icing on the cake – it is one of the most important and binding of the basic ingredients.' Even the Catholic Church recognizes non-consummation as one of the few grounds for nullifying a marriage, and there is an old saying that the rocks on which a marriage breaks up are usually to be found in the bed. So what can you do when, as the perennially active rock star of the Rolling Stones, Mick Jagger, sings, you *'can't get no satisfaction?'*

Is it your age?

Although most people assume that sexual activity is likely to decrease with age, in the swinging sixties the experts gave a different picture. They, together with more recent investigators, found that sexual interest and morning erections, good markers for either actual or potential erectile power, declined very gradually with age and only went below the 50 percent mark when men hit their nineties. The actual frequency of sexual intercourse dropped away much more rapidly, however, and reached the 50 percent mark at around 70, mainly due to erectile failure.[1]

Shakespeare recognized this problems 400 years ago when he wrote, *'Is it not strange that desire should so many years outlive performance?'* This question taxes the minds of doctors and their patients to this day.

The answer could well be that lower levels of testosterone are needed to maintain libido than are required for potency. There are also many complex circulatory factors involved in obtaining an erection as well as in the hormonal drive. The spirit is still willing, often long after the flesh has weakened, although following repeated erectile failure, the desire also tends to fade eventually. It is difficult to assess what is essentially physical and what is psychological, a combination of expectations, attitude and monogamy leading to monotony.

These problems are likely to grow as more women go on long-term HRT at menopause. In such cases the big drop in sexual interest and enjoyment which was well documented for women in their fifties has declined or even been reversed. Yet this is just the time when andropausal men are experiencing the biggest decline in both libido and potency. So women's expectations of continuing sexual activity are rising year by year and men are literally not able to keep up with them. Increasingly, couples are likely to get sexually out of step, particularly as men tend to marry women a few years younger than themselves, with the male lagging further and further behind.

A loving sexual relationship is not only enjoyable, though, but can actually keep you young. Evidence from a recent study by Dr David Weeks, a clinical neuropsychologist at the Edinburgh Royal Infirmary, suggests that the aging process can be delayed by making love more than twice a week. He recruited a group of people in Europe and America who claimed to look and feel much younger than they actually were and got them to send him their photos and fill in a lifestyle questionnaire. He also asked a control group from the same part of each country to do the same and then got independent assessors to guess the age of all 3,500 people, who ranged in age from their twenties to over 100.

The results were clear cut; the youthful test group were rated 12 to 14 years on average younger than they actually were and the control group one or two years younger. The differences on the questionnaire were even more striking, the 'young lovers' having sex much more often than their peers, and many, both men and women, having much younger partners. However, an important feature of any relationship was that it was a loving and happy one.

This is similar to the results on factors which prevent coronary heart disease. A group in the Netherlands showed that feeling loved was one of the most important things that kept heart trouble away. As Woody Allen says, '*Love is the answer, but sex raises some interesting questions.*' Perhaps if we can answer some of these questions, the loving element will have a greater chance to express itself.

Sexual chemistry

Testosterone is the hormone which largely regulates desire in both men and women, although its levels are generally 10 to 20 times higher in the male. It is thought to act both directly on the brain, and indirectly in making the genital areas more sensitive and responsive, also enlarging the penis or clitoris. Thus it is generally a sexual stimulant for both sexes.

Experience with patients and research reviewed by Professor Bancroft of the Medical Research Council Reproductive Biology Unit in Edinburgh in his book *Human Sexuality and its Problems* suggest that there is less overlap between the laboratory 'normal range' of testosterone and its 'behaviorally relevant range' in men than in women.[2] This means that if the laboratory measures testosterone levels in 100 'normal' men, age and sexual activity often unspecified, in 95 percent, values of, say, 10-30 nmol/l may be recorded. Many studies, including my own, have shown that the libido will be increased by testosterone treatment in men whose values lie in the range 5-15 nmol/l, although the proportion of free, biologically active hormone is, as emphasized elsewhere, also very important.

However, in women, the 'normal range' is only 1-2 nmol/l, but libido may go on rising up to 70-10 nmol/l or even higher. This is shown after giving testosterone treatment, both orally and by pellet implant, to those suffering lack of desire or who have lost their ability to have an orgasm for no obvious psychological reason. It is also reported in women self-medicating with very high doses of testosterone, either in athletes or those wishing to become 'The Third Sex' (see page 40).

That the level of free, biologically active testosterone is vital to libido in both sexes and sexual function in the male is shown by studies on epileptics. Anti-epilepsy drugs raise the sex hormone binding globulin protein, holding the testosterone in the blood and preventing it acting.[3] Both the libido and morning erections are reduced while patients take these drugs, but when they come off them, the binding protein levels fall, their testosterone is freed up again and the libido and morning erections are restored.[4] This is a perfect model of male menopause and conclusively demonstrates its reversibility.

The science of sexual attraction

Poets and songwriters have mused for millennia why it is that people fall in love. Psychologists and pharmacologists may now have cracked the problem between them. Although their results may not immediately improve their love life or ours, they offer hope for an understanding.

The psychologists have discovered the effects of early imprinting and bonding which occur at birth and in infancy. The newborn child is not the passive plastic doll it was once thought to be, but a highly receptive, rapidly developing, sentient being. It is aware of, responds to and learns from the complex inputs from all its faculties. Even in the subdued pink gloom of the womb it is thought to be soothed by the rhythmic beating of the mother's heart, the whooshing of the blood flowing in her abdominal vessels and the inner reverberations of her voice.

At birth, it is catapulted into the blinding light of a chilly operating theater, held upside down and slapped until it cries as its mother screams with the pain of childbirth. In the best of natural childbirth practices, although hi tech help is at hand if needed, the child is immediately reunited with its mother, held lovingly in her arms, and gazes through the accurately fixed focus of its eyes at her face, listening to her soft and gentle voice. In the first few minutes and hours afterward, like all mammals, there is a complex emotional and physical bonding process involving all the senses, which will last for life. If this goes well, it can lay firm foundations for emotional stability throughout childhood and adult life. If it is disrupted by separation, illness or emotional or physical trauma to mother or child, it can leave lasting psychological damage.

It is probable that the variations and mishaps which occur in this bonding process leave the corresponding small or large psychological scars which decide whether and how we are going to bond from puberty onward. After all, dogs separated from their mothers in the first few hours or days of life and weaned by humans, often seem to assume they are human and relate more to human beings than they do to other dogs. The biologist Konrad Lorenz first reported how geese he held immediately after hatching and fed for the first few days of life became imprinted on him and for the rest of their lives waddled after him, convinced they were eminent biologists. Cygnets similarly reared by a cameraman would follow him anywhere, whether he was walking, in a car or in a boat. As fully grown birds they could then be trained to carry light cameras on their backs and achieve beautiful films of formations of swans in flight from literally a bird's eye view.

With models like this, is it any wonder that men tend to fall in love with women who resemble their mothers, either in their looks, the tone of their voices or possibly even the way they smell?

Pheromones

Even more than by sight and sound, throughout the animal kingdom, Cupid's arrows are carried by bodily scents. Timeless examples include dogs seeking out a bitch in heat, the musk ox scenting a potential mate miles away and the stallion that catches the scent of the mare. Although perfumes were developed thousands of years ago mainly to cover up unpleasant body odors with more attractive ones, the more skilled perfumiers learned from the ability of animals to smell and be sexually attracted by the opposite sex before they catch sight of them.

The term 'pheromone' was coined by the German biochemist Adolf Butenandt in 1959 and was another of his major contributions to science, the first being his discovery and synthesis of testosterone nearly 25 years previously (see page 16). The term is derived from the Greek *phero* ('to carry') and *hormao* ('to excite'.) This is an apt description of these airborne chemical messages promising sexual excitement, a sort of long-range biological dating agency.

Although first described in female silkworm moths, pheromones were also found in female monkeys and in women, where they peaked at ovulation and were under the control of estrogen. Thus it was shown that from the time when estrogens surged at puberty, the inner female hormones started the production of these outer chemical signs of sexual maturity and availability.

The main sex hormone in men, the androgen testosterone, acts similarly. It is broken down into two components called androstenone and androstenol, which at a subliminal level are thought to be powerful sexual attractants. They are released in the odors of the armpits and scrotum, in urine and in saliva. Androstenone gives a characteristic smell to male urine and is what the sow is detecting when snuffling for truffles, which is perhaps why this rare and exotic fungus has a reputation for being an aphrodisiac. Androstenol has a musky odor, which is less obvious, but probably equally potent.

As the average female nose is at the height of the average male armpit, dancing can be seen as an intense form of exchange of bodily scents preceding the exchange of bodily fluids.

After andropause, because of the low testosterone levels, the phermonally deprived male does not feel as sexy or smell as sexy as the pungent, sexually active man in his prime. Research urgently needs to be done to see whether pheromones are restored by hormone replacement therapy with the parent compound, testosterone.

Ready for love

Why is it that in spring a young man's fancy lightly turns to thoughts of love? Well, even though the mating season isn't what it used to be, probably because of all year-round stimulation by artificial lighting and television, there are good reasons for this in terms of the hormonal rites of spring.

As the urban cave dweller emerges blinking into the spring sunshine, he drinks up the sun. This is seen particularly in the more northern countries such as Scandinavia, where the winter nights are long and the days often overcast with clouds. There people often just sit out in the open sunning themselves as though mentally thawing out.

As already explained, the bright light and lengthening days have the effect of reducing the level of melatonin, the 'hibernation hormone.' Some people seem to get a surge of this hormone in the autumn and it makes them feel quite torpid and depressed, a condition known as seasonal affective disorder, or SAD for short. This can be prevented or treated by midwinter sunshine holidays or by bursts of intense artificial daylight.

In spring, the reduction in the production of melatonin not only generally causes greater mental alertness, but also raises levels of a variety of brain chemicals, called neurotransmitters, which stimulate and arouse us, making us full of the joys of spring.

Because these neurotransmitters regulate mood, they have been the target for intensive study by most of the major pharmaceutical companies, who see the potential market for the chemical production of happiness, peace and love in bottled form. Aldous Huxley, in his book *Brave New World* back in the 1920s, first coined the advertising slogan for the mythical drug 'Soma' of *'Take a gram and don't give a damn.'* Unfortunately since then there have been many false dawns. The prototypic tranquilizer Valium was originally marketed with pictures of tigers changing into pussycats. In the same way, some of the early antidepressant drugs showed pictures of space rockets lifting off for the moon to illustrate the hoped for lifting of the spirits. However, although they have proved useful in some cases of severe depression, the results have often been somewhat depressing to patients and doctors alike. Unfortunately it has been found that if you take the edge off the 'razor blade of life down which we slide,' according to the American humorist Tom Lehrer, you also take the edge off many of life's joys and blunt performance and creativity.

So it seems that the complex mysteries of the human brain still elude our grasp. Although advances in psychopharmacology are steadily improving the drugs available for mental ailments, we cannot safely manipulate mood without risking severe side effects. We have been able to get to the Sea of Tranquility on the moon, but still come back to a sea of tranquilizers on the Earth.

Unfortunately, it is in the field of sexual activity that the undesirable side effects of tranquilizers, antidepressants and sleeping pills are most severe and unpleasant. For liveliness, loving, libido and the pursuit of sexual fulfilment, we need just the right mixture of hormones and neurotransmitters, in the right brain cells, at the right rime. Drug treatments are at present very hit and miss. This is why unless anxiety and/or depression are very severe and prolonged it is generally better to use gentle non drug approaches such as psychotherapy and psychosexual counseling – meditation rather than medication.

The food of love

There are some foods which may gently enhance both desire and sexual activity, through regulating brain chemistry.

Two of the most important neurotransmitters in the brain are serotonin and the monoamines. Serotonin is derived from a plasma amino acid called tryptophan and after this is taken up into the brain, a good supply of vitamin B_6 is needed for its conversion. Most diets contain sufficient protein to supply the necessary tryptophan and too much protein may increase competition from other amino acids for uptake into the brain. these competing amino acids can be removed by the release of insulin, so simple sugars such as glucose and sucrose, which produce this, will improve the uptake of tryptophan and hence the production of serotonin.

The predominant brain monoamine is noradrenaline. It is produced in the brain, again with the help of vitamin B6, from the amino acid tyrosine. This is also present in most proteins and is easily taken up into the brain in proportion to the amount of protein in the diet.

Another monoamine is phenylethylamine, which is present in chocolate and may account for its reputed aphrodisiac properties.

Armed with all this essential biochemical information, we can concoct a meal almost guaranteed to stimulate passion. After the relaxing champagne, which also stimulates female testosterone production, we have the suggestive goat's cheese starter, redolent with monoamines. This is followed by the minute steak, to boost tyrosine, new potatoes with butter, again to help testosterone production, and a fresh green salad to enhance vitamin C levels. The *coup de grâce* is the 'death by chocolate' cake, topped with B_6-rich walnuts. This is surely a recipe for sexual success, providing it doesn't bring on a splitting migraine headache in the woman or an instant heart attack in the man.

Can sexual satisfaction be improved?

Certainly it is possible in the vast majority of andropausal cases to improve sexual satisfaction for both partners, not only by TRT, but also by a range of additional techniques such as sex education, focusing particularly on the physical, hormonal and emotional changes occurring in the male, and, where necessary, psychosexual counseling or marital therapy. With reassurance that there may be a physical basis for the male partner's apparent lack of desire, as well as his unwillingness or inability to perform, a tense situation can often be defused and the relationship helped on the road to recovery.

In particular, emphasizing the good nonsexual areas of the relationship and the enjoyment that both partners get from them can reduce the friction. One or both may also need to learn a good relaxation technique, as described in Chapter 9, and small amounts of alcohol, such as a shared bottle of wine, can help.

For most couples, when the first flush of passion is over, a sexual session needs time and energy. Erections are more difficult for a man to maintain when he is rushed or tired or both. If one or both partners are under pressure, a 'dating' system may help when they choose a time and place when they feel most relaxed and happiest together. One patient, when I suggested this, said he and his wife had such different conflicting time deadlines in their busy lives that it was like timing a moon shot. If it works, however, by some mysterious process it usually gets easier and easier to find time for these love-making sessions.

Massage, especially in subdued light or candlelight, and with music to soothe the savage breast, can be both relaxing and a turn on, as well as being part of 'getting in touch.' Giving kind, loving and encouraging comments to the other person and the effect they are having on you, works much better than even the most constructive criticism. Fortunately, nature is kind in that we tend to get farsighted around the age of 50, so that skin blemishes and the occasional wrinkle are blurred, and hopefully we remember how our partners looked in their physical prime.

Such methods are all part of encouraging the realization that sexual activity can be pleasant and satisfying even without penetration. Usually under sufficiently relaxed conditions both partners can have orgasms by mutual masturbation, oral sex or any of the increasing variety of 'sex-aids' that can be bought by mail order or from a sex shop. Sexy garments, perhaps chosen by the other person, also have their part to play in setting the scene.

Fortunately, with the more frank approach that medical assessment and treatment encourages, combined with these common sense self-help measures, the situation usually improves to the point where full intercourse resumes or becomes more satisfying. If this doesn't happen and there still appears to be anxiety or an emotional part to the problem, then a more gradual approach under the guidance of a properly qualified sex therapist should be tried. The therapist will often advise a technique known as 'sensate focus,' which involves stages of being touched for your own pleasure without genital contact, then giving feedback on what you find enjoyable as well as unpleasant, and finally enjoying the experience of touching and being touched, including genital contact and, if it happens, orgasm, although this is not the aim.

Premature ejaculation, which often accompanies erectile difficulties, can be treated by medication, as described later, or by a 'stop-start' technique, initially by hand, and then with the woman sitting astride the man to give better control of withdrawal and re-entry.[5] Alternatively, the 'squeeze' method, described originally by Masters and Johnson in 1970,[6] can be used. Here, when the man is about to ejaculate, the woman gently but firmly squeezes the base of the head of the penis until the impulse to ejaculate subsides.

One worrying statistic is that in a community-based study, just over half of the male subjects aged between 40 and 70, felt that their erections were inadequate. This is also the most common problem men present in male sexual dysfunction clinics and it peaks at the time when andropause appears, that is the mid-forties onward.[7] This is a major health problem which is seldom adequately investigated or treated. So at this stage it is appropriate to describe how erections happen so that we can better understand what can go wrong, especially with age or an insufficient hormonal head of steam, and how to help.

The mechanics of erection

Man's ability to have an erection, which has been worshipped from the earliest of times, is actually a recurring miracle of hydraulic engineering. It is brought about by a complex series of chemical changes and nerve reflexes, which work together to increase the amount of blood flowing into the penis and temporarily decrease the amount going out. Two elongated blood sacs, the *corpora cavernosa*, become engorged and create the erection. This event, which is achieved with effortless and sometimes embarrassing ease in the teens and twenties, usually becomes a more difficult feat in the thirties and forties, can be variable in the fifties and sixties, and is often a disappointingly brief and infrequent wonder in the seventies and beyond, especially in the 'hormonally challenged' andropausal male.

For the amount of blood going into the penis to be adequate for an erection, there needs to be a good flow of blood in the artery to the penis, relaxation of the blood vessels inside it and reduction of the amount of blood draining out. It is like pumping up a bicycle tire and hoping for a smooth ride. If you don't pump hard enough, if the walls of the inner tube are weak or stuck together, or if the valve is leaky and lets the air out as fast as it goes in, only hopes are inflated.

Sometimes the small artery supplying blood to the penis is clogged up because of a generalized arterial degeneration called atheromatosis, which is the most common cause of coronary heart disease. This is more frequent in those with high blood cholesterol levels, in diabetics and in smokers, who are more prone to erection problems. Fortunately, it is seldom sufficient on its own to cause the problem, and when it is, arterial surgery to provide additional blood supply is occasionally successful.

The pooling of blood in the penis which produces its rigidity is dependent on hormonal priming, local chemical factors and a balance of nerve stimulation. Because of the complexity of this mechanism, it is easily upset by hormonal insufficiency, a wide range of medications and emotional reactions, especially anxiety. Each of these needs to be considered in cases of erectile difficulty and corrected where possible. Often the efforts of the patient and his partner to overcome the problem are just as important as the doctor's.

The story seems appropriate here of the man who went to seek medical advice and was given treatment which required him to make a lot of lifestyle changes. Being by nature a lazy fellow, before he left the doctor's office he asked the white-coated man sitting behind the desk with disbelief, *'Are you a real doctor?'*

'The question is,' replied the doctor, *'are you a real patient?'*

Testosterone and erectile function

Although it is difficult to say precisely what part testosterone plays in helping to produce erections, it certainly both primes the penis and triggers the chain of events which bring an erection about. It is surprising but gratifying how often when adequate testosterone therapy is given, all the symptoms of andropause disappear within a few weeks or months, including erectile difficulties, particularly when other factors contributing to its onset or continuation are dealt with. A statistically significant improvement in erectile function occurred in over 70 percent of my first 1,000 cases treated with a variety of different forms of testosterone. This was particularly marked with the more powerful oral preparation, Restandol, which sometimes needed to be given in high but safe doses, and with the pellet implants.

Although this use of testosterone to help erection problems is controversial and not acknowledged by some authorities, this is certainly not my experience in this large group of patients. The efficiency of testosterone in restoring potency is a common experience with doctors prepared to give it an adequate trial. It was even recognized over 50 years ago in the article on the 'male climacteric' by Drs Heller and Myers described in detail in the first chapter of this book (see pages 18–20). They found that erectile function returned in nearly all of their testosterone deficient patients when they gave the hormone and went away again when they stopped.[8]

Even though it is more difficult to restore function than desire, unless the source of the problems is obviously psychological, it seems logical to investigate the level of free active testosterone and boost it if it is low. If nothing else, the accompanying increases in libido, confidence and energy will greatly encourage the patient to try supplementary medicinal methods, if needed.

Sexercise

Sex is the most vigorous form of exercise most people do, and for some it is the only form. Measurements of pulse rate, blood pressure and hormones before, during and afterward have shown surges in the stress hormones during sexual activity, together with rises in heart rate and blood pressure. Fortunately, these go down to baseline levels or even below in the recovery phase afterward, and there is then an increase in testosterone in both sexes.

For this reason, regular sexual activity, even if the man cannot always achieve penetration, is to be encouraged in the prevention and treatment of andropause. If this is not possible, either because a partner is not available or not willing, then masturbation about once a week stops the erectile system 'going rusty,' and may stimulate testosterone production. As Woody Allen says, '*At least masturbation is sex with someone you love.*'

Drugs which help and drugs which hinder

Drugs given for medical reasons can often play a part in bringing on the erectile problems which contribute to menopause. The motto is, 'If in doubt, check it out.'

Virtually any drug used to reduce blood pressure, but especially diuretics and the so called beta blockers, can be a problem here.[9] Because hypertension is often stress related and not so much an illness as a way of life, stress management techniques can be tried to control mild to moderate elevations in blood pressure (see pages 168–71). Reduced stress will also help to reduce the performance anxiety element in erection problems.

Alternatively, sometimes switching to a different medicine, such as Labetolol (Tranxene) or the new 'alpha-blockers,' such as doxazosin (Cardura) which seem to interfere less with erections, can be helpful in combination with testosterone treatment. TRT does not itself generally raise blood pressure and may in some cases lower it.

A wide variety of tranquilizers and antidepressants are also associated with impaired erections. These are used to treat many conditions with symptoms which overlap with those of menopause, so it is often not clear which is doing what.[10] Virtually all antidepressants can have a harmful effect, except possibly the newer generation of drugs such as Prozac. Prozac is occasionally helpful in treating depression associated with andropause and it also seems to reduce the common tendency to premature ejaculation which accompanies difficulty in maintaining an erection.

The newer compounds have a different action on the brain from those used to treat depression, by inhibiting the uptake of a chemical by which one brain cell activates another, 5 hydroxy-tryptamine (5HT). Some specialists are sufficiently enthusiastic about this type of compound to recommend its use in premature ejaculation, although through limited experience this may prove to be a case of premature ejudication. An antidepressant called Venlafaxine (Efexor) made by

Wyeth is reputed to have the least effect on libido or erectile function and few side effects generally.

Another possible exception is the older antidepressant Trasadone, marketed in the UK as Molypaxin. Given as a single dose of 75 to 150 mg half an hour before sex, it can in some cases help in obtaining erections over a one or two hour period. Its effectiveness varies widely from person to person and it may just make them feel sleepy, which is not usually the desired effect.

Asthma treatments such as ephedrine and many other inhalers can also sometimes make erection problems worse, and a trial of withdrawing or switching treatment where possible can help.

Even stomach medicines such as Tagamet have infrequently been shown to cause problems, as have a seemingly endless list of medicines.[11]

Drugs of addiction appear only to be a problem if used in large amounts, causing psychological or social problems. They may, however, accompany an alcohol problem, or be used to avoid facing up to the issues contributing to andropause. The appropriate agencies such as Narcotics Anonymous may need to be involved here. The most common drug of addiction, nicotine, can also be a threat to potency and for this and many other health reasons is best avoided. It has been found that one cigarette can temporarily halve penile blood flow. Although smoking once had a sexy image, we now understand why macho film stars are only seen smoking *after* sex scenes, or else a long time before.

Although erection problems often decrease or even disappear with combined treatment with testosterone and the other measures described, there may be some continuing difficulty, particularly in diabetics or those with heart and circulatory problems. In such cases, there are a range of other measures which can usually solve the problem one way or another.

Yohimbine, marketed as Yocon, is a medicine from the bark of an African tree, *Pausinystalia yohimbe*, which when taken by mouth, in some cases seems to act on the brain as a sexual stimulant, both boosting the libido and improving erections, particularly in people on testosterone. It seems to have a good effect when taken as one 5 mg pill each morning on a regular basis. Yohimbine shouldn't be given to nervous individuals, who can become more anxious on it, or those with high blood pressure, where it can have an unpredictable effect.

There are also various substances which can be injected into the penis by the patient himself just before intercourse to provide a serviceable and sustained erection. Many men find it a bit cold-blooded and premeditated, and their partners find it unromantic, mechanical and sometimes an insult to their sex appeal. As one wife said, inaccurately in her husband's case, *'If I were as attractive as Marilyn Monroe, he would get an erection immediately, wouldn't he?'* So, although this treatment has a high success rate, with usually around two thirds of even resistant cases responding, about half the people who say they'll try it drop out because they or their partners find it unacceptable.

Papaverine is the most commonly used of these injections, and is a cheap and stable preparation. It is injected through a short and very fine needle into the shaft of the penis, and increases the flow of blood into the two spongy *corpora cavernosa*, helping to produce and maintain an erection. According to the carefully regulated amount injected from the small syringe provided, which is similar to that used by diabetics, the length of time the erection is maintained can be adjusted, according to taste and joint enthusiasm of the partners, from 15 minutes to one hour or more. Moreover, it continues even after the man has reached orgasm and ejaculated, which some couples find adds to their enjoyment.

Apart from its artificiality, there are other drawbacks to this treatment, however. The slight stinging pain experienced when the needle is jabbed into this very sensitive part of the male anatomy and the possibility of bruising, especially if the patient is on anticoagulants or even aspirin, can put some men off. Also, sometimes erections persist for several hours or more, which can be dangerous as well as uncomfortable and socially inconvenient. If an erection lasts for more than four hours, it is known medically as priapism. This should be dealt with as soon as possible in a hospital emergency department to avoid bruising which may last days, if not weeks.

More gentle in its action and less liable to cause priapism is the injection of alprostadil, a medication similar to the natural substance in the body called prostaglandin E1. The medication is called Caverject and is manufactured by Upjohn Pharmaceuticals. This is a definite advance, but tends to cost about the same as a bottle of champagne for each shot, and even if you can afford the expense, unlike champagne, it is not recommended for use more than three times a week.

There is also a tiny pellet of alprostodil, which can be inserted into the opening of the urethra at the tip of the penis, and is rapidly absorbed into the *corpora cavernosa*. The system known as MUSE (Medicated Urethral System for Erection) is made by VIVUS in the USA, and marketed by Astra in Europe. As described in the next chapter, these preparations containing the expensive and difficult to administer hormone Alprostadil have largely been replaced by oral medication, especially Viagra.

Mechanical methods

There are various mechanical devices which can be used to promote the flow of blood into the penis and lessen the amount going out. The simplest of these is a rubber ring, usually called the Blako ring, which comes in different sizes and, when rolled down the semierect penis, reduces the outflow of blood in the veins, which can help to obtain and maintain a full erection.

Another aid is a suction device consisting of a glass tube which is slipped over the penis and applies negative pressure gently to it by means of a mechanical pump (Erectaid). When a full erection has been achieved, a tight rubber band similar to the Blako ring is slipped off the end of the tube nearest the patient and prevents the blood in the penis from flowing away. However, many men find this way of getting an erection cumbersome, unromantic and even painful, so it leaves a lot to be desired.

Surgical techniques

Rarely, none of these treatments or the new oral agents work and then the opinion of a urologist specializing in this field should be sought. After investigation of the arterial inflow and venous outflow of the penis, they may recommend vascular surgery, or one of the inflatable or soft metal, 'bendy-toy' penile implants. All these methods can produce good results in the right hands, but none of them is much use if the other symptoms of menopause, especially lack of libido, are untreated.

Good times coming

There have been important new developments recently in the field of nitric oxide and the erectile mechanism. A new type of nerve has recently been discovered in many organs in the body, including the penis, which, among other important actions, relaxes the smooth muscle fibers controlling the diameter of small blood vessels. These are known as 'nitrurgic' nerves because by releasing nitric oxide they allow the blood vessels in the penis to dilate and then become engorged with blood, producing an erection.

Anything that helps nitric oxide production or activity, encourages the erection. Amyl nitrate has been used for sexual stimulation, as well as its ability to relax smooth muscle in various parts of the body.

Pharmacologists have, as you can imagine, been working around the clock to synthesize a drug which would prolong the action of nitric oxide. One topical application, in both senses of the word, is a cream which, when applied to the shaft of the penis half an hour before inter-course, is absorbed through the skin, causing engorgement of the *corpora cavernosa*, so that erection is greatly helped. A very well conducted and encouraging trial of this pharmacological cocktail was recently reported in the *British Medical Journal* article by an Egyptian professor, Adel Gomaa.[12]

As far as oral preparations go, at present the drug company Pfizer appears to be ahead of the field. It has come up with a drug taken by mouth which helps nitric oxide to work, so that its active agents accumulate in the walls of the penile blood vessels, keeping them relaxed and the penis erect. This is Viagra, also known as sildenafil, and for reasons explained in the next chapter, in the field of erection problems is truly a breakthrough drug.

Chapter eight

Viagra and the magic gun

Most men dream of having a magic gun – one that rises to any occasion, is ready for instant action any time they want to use it, has perfect aim and can be sure to fire not just once, but several times, if needed.

This is the James Bond-like image that links gun and penis ... Kiss – Kiss, Bang – Bang. It is not just the phallocentric fantasy in Ian Fleming stories but the shared imagery of men and women, equating potency and power, desire and sexual satisfaction. Bond can shoot his manly way to the heart of the villain's woman, and save the world in his spare time. Sex sirens like Mae West ask their suitors, 'Is that a gun in your pocket, or are you just glad to see me?'

Mother Nature, alas, had other plans. She invented sex for procreation rather than recreation, and when a man was past his reproductive shelf life, she all too often disarmed him. This is especially the case now that women taking Hormone Replacement Therapy are experiencing 'Post-Menopausal Zest.' They are preserving their vitality and attractiveness, together with their expectations of an active sex life into their fifties, sixties and even seventies and beyond. What was regarded only as an occupational hazard for aging rakes and roués has become a commonplace problem for the majority of men in middle age and later life.

This decline in potency was well described as long ago as 1925 by one of the longest standing, if that is the right word, of sexual gymnasts, the writer Frank Harris. In his five volume autobiography, 'My Life and Loves,' he describes his decrease in firepower with age.[1]

'My Creator – when I was wholly without experience and had only just entered my teens, gave me, so to speak, a magazine gun of sex, and hardly had I learned its use and enjoyment when he took it away from me forever, and gave me in its place a double-barreled gun: after a few years, he took that away and gave me a single-barreled gun with which I was forced to content myself for the best part of my life.

'Towards the end the old single-barrel began to show signs of wear and age: sometimes it would go off too soon, sometimes it missed fire and shamed me, do what I would.

'I want to teach youths how to use their magazine gun of sex so that it may last for years, and when they come to the double-barrel, how to take such care that the good weapon will do them liege service right into their fifties, and the single-barrel will then give them pleasure up to three score years and ten.'

In his later writings, Harris records that for him the end not just of potency, but even desire, was the beginning of death: there was nothing else to live for. This suggests that well into later life, next to a fear of death, men fear impotence. However, impotence is an imprecise term and probably better expressed as 'erectile dysfunction,' or even just 'erection problems' of varying degrees of severity.

Men performing badly

Experts can't even agree on a definition of impotence – Does it mean failure 50 percent of the time, a crucial point where performance anxiety sets in? Or is it just the official definition of 'inability to achieve an erection satisfactory for intercourse?'

The size of the problem, and hence the market for drugs to treat it, is enormous. As men tend to deny it, like an iceberg, only 10 percent shows on the surface and arrives in the doctor's office for treatment. This is shown in several studies in America and the UK over the last ten years.

America – Massachusetts Male Aging Study[2]

This very detailed and extensive study published in 1993 interviewed a random sample of over 1,700 men aged 40–70 who had been asked about their potency over the previous six months. The most common complaint with increasing age was 'moderate impotence,' defined as a problem attaining or maintaining an erection 50 percent of the time. Half of the men over 40 had experienced some degree of impotence, and from these figures it was estimated that of 40 million males in this age group in the US in 1994, 19 million were likely to have significant problems with erections. Allowing for aging of the population, this was likely to rise to 30 million in 1998 and 54 million in 2010, truly an epidemic of erection problems.

Great Britain

A MORI survey on 'Men, Health and Sex' carried out in 1993 inquired about erectile function in a random sample of 802 'Older Men.' Half of the sexually active men complained of poor erections since they turned 50. Nearly a third of the men over the age of 50 said they NEVER have sexual intercourse any more.

Viagra – a giant leap for mankind

In the treatment of erectile dysfunction (E.D.), Viagra is 'a giant leap for mankind.' Probably more men care about putting the manhood back in the man than putting a man on the moon. In fact, this drug can put a man and woman over the moon by ending the dreaded ED and the misery this causes.

Viagra seems to have caught the public's imagination just as much as the media's attention. Not even NASA's triumphal moon landing equalled Viagra in terms of publicity by making the cover of the two American magazines, Time and Business Week, simultaneously.

Does it deserve this degree of hype? There are compelling reasons for believing it does, both as a major advance in a long neglected area of men's health, and as the official dawn of a 'New Era of Lifestyle Drugs.'

Then there was Viagra

This 'Wonder Drug' hit the headlines as soon as it was launched on the American market, receiving FDA approval on March 27th, 1998, an historic day. Indeed, like a marketing man's dream, it has been in the news on and off ever since. For doctors treating ED, and the large majority of patients suffering from it, there have been two stages in their condition: 'Before Viagra (BV)' and 'After Viagra (AV).' Let's have a look at the sequence of events for the three months around the launch of Viagra before we consider whether events have born out the high hopes for this drug:

Sunday London Times: March 22nd –
Male sex pill poised to raise American hopes and 'Impotence Inc' profits – The male equivalent of the Wonderbra. – Sales of $300M predicted for the rest of the year.

New York Times: March 28th –
U.S. approves sale of impotence pill: Huge market seen – 70 percent of patients helped – 30 million U.S. males affected – 50 percent of all men aged 40–70.

International Herald Tribune: March 30th –
Baby boomers will be willing to spend money to have their lives enhanced. For right now, the men's market has moved in front of the women's.
The market for satisfying male complaints – especially impotence – is largely untapped. Of estimated 30m with the problem, only 2.76m visited doctors about it last year.

Times: April 4th –
Impotence pill could be on offer this year – 'Whether Viagra will be prescribed on the NHS remains to be seen.' Unsure 'How much drug-assisted sex is reasonable.' 'High potential for inappropriate use' foreseen.

Time Magazine: May 4th –

Cover picture story about 'The Potency Pill' says 'Yes, VIAGRA works! And the craze says a lot about men, women and sex.'

Business Week Magazine: May 11th –

Cover picture story about 'VIAGRA: The New Era of Lifestyle Drugs.' 'Pfizer's impotence pill is more than just a blockbuster drug to treat a specific medical problem. It will also enhance the quality of life for "healthy" people. Similar drugs lie ahead: for anxiety, weight problems, memory loss, and symptoms of aging. In the process, the $300 billion drug industry will be transformed.'

Previously there had been gradual advances in the war against erection problems, but Viagra revolutionized this entire area of treatment, largely making the other remedies obsolete.

This was dramatically shown during a meeting I attended of leading UK experts on erection problems held in central London on May 14th, 1998. We sat around all morning discussing the theoretical benefits of different types of erection treatments and ways they might be marketed. At lunch-time someone dashed in with faxed copies of the first large-scale study of the effectiveness of Viagra which had been published in the *New England Journal of Medicine* that morning.[3] There was shocked silence as we sat and read the huge amount of evidence in the article for Viagra being the safest, most effective and most easily applied form of treatment. As far as we were concerned, that was game, set and match to Viagra, and after quitting early, the group never met again. How had this major advance been made?

Dr NO – the nitric oxide story

The whole subject of nitric oxide and its many important actions in the body is a very exciting and 'sexy' area of medical research, in every sense of the word. It was only just over ten years ago that some of its many roles were first discovered, and already it is the target for a billion dollar pharmaceutical arms race.

The title of Dr NO should rightfully go to Professor Salvador Moncada. He was the British research biologist who discovered that nitric oxide (NO) was actually being produced within the human body and had a range of very important actions, not least of which was playing a crucial role in producing erections. Over the last decade the image of nitric oxide has changed from being just another toxic pollutant of car exhausts to a key transmitter in a whole new nervous system, regulating blood flow, asthma attacks and the immune system.

Professor Moncada, like most great innovators, made his great discovery using the usual mixture of 1 percent inspiration and 99 percent perspiration. He had been working for several years on the theory that there must be two types of nerves controlling the size of small arteries and regulating the flow of blood through them. One type was called noradrenergic, because the nerve endings in the muscle wall released the hormone noradrenaline (norepinephrine) which constricted the artery. It had been known for many years that if this system was acting in many parts of the body it could increase blood pressure. What Prof. Moncada was searching for was a totally different kind of nerve, releasing a different chemical messenger, which would relax blood vessels, let more blood flow through them, and drop blood pressure.

Nitrates had been used for many years to dilate the coronary arteries, and relieve the pain of insufficient blood going to the heart, called angina. The experts agreed that the active ingredient of these drugs, nitric oxide, wasn't produced naturally in the body. Prof. Moncada thought otherwise, but of course had to prove it against fierce opposition from all the other pharmacologists in the field.

His reasoned that the substance he was seeking was produced by the inner lining of the blood vessel, the endothelium. He called this the 'Endothelium Derived Relaxing Factor' (EDRF), and found with elegant experiments on small sections of animal arteries suspended in water baths, that if you removed this lining, you could make the vessel constrict but not relax.

Then he had to find out what was being released from this lining, and prove the identity of EDRF. He started by showing that it had the same biological properties as nitric oxide through a range of experiments using low concentrations of the highly purified gas, which had to be freshly made as it was very unstable.[4]

The next problem was that although relatively large amounts of nitric oxide, in the exhaust fumes of cars for example, could be measured by a detector using a technique called chemiluminescence, a far more sensitive method was needed to demonstrate it in individual cells. He therefore developed a special technique of studying endothelial cells grown on cover glass and examining them under the microscope before and after stimulation with substances which were thought to cause nitric oxide release. You can imagine the excitement in the laboratory when the dancing, blue-staining, nitric oxide gas particles could finally be seen under the microscope.[5] The nerves which caused this release of the gas were termed 'nitrurgic nerves' and they were rapidly identified in blood vessels and other tissues all over the body, in the brain, eye, heart, lungs, gut, and, last but not least, in the penis.

Suddenly, the walls of entrenched medical dogma came tumbling down, and researchers from every discipline saw how it could affect the medical treatment in their specialty. Cardiologists, respiratory physicians, immunologists and even doctors treating toxic shock all woke up to the fact that this was something they needed to know about and to think how that knowledge could be used to derive treatments in their field.

In 1992 nitric oxide was voted 'Molecule of the Year' by *Science* magazine. Publication rates of articles in medical journals about nitric oxide have risen from virtually zero to over ten thousand a year. From a few brief paragraphs in medical toxicology books, there are now many textbooks and even a seven volume series devoted to the latest research in this rapidly expanding universe of new knowledge. Over five hundred publications later however, Professor Moncada still holds the title of Dr NO.

Magic molecule to magic gun

One obvious use of this magic molecule was to try to dilate the coronary arteries carrying blood to the heart muscle where they were furred up and causing the severe chest pain of angina. Dr Ian Osterloh, a research scientist at Pfizer's UK laboratory at Sandwich in Kent, set up a study of a newly produced drug called sildenafil citrate, which is the chemical name for Viagra. This was known to promote nitric oxide production by inhibiting an enzyme, phosphodiesterase, which rapidly breaks down the nitric oxide being produced by the endothelial cells which relaxes the blood vessels.

Fortunately, as it turned out, the drug trial was not a great success, and the patients got little relief from their angina. What fascinated Dr Osterloh however, was that when the trial was stopped because it was not having much effect on the coronary arteries, the patients were curiously reluctant to return their unused supplies of pills. When he asked the patients why this was, he was told that although it didn't help their chest pain much, it did wonders for their erections, sometimes restoring them after years of impotence. He was quick to realize that the sildenafil was specific for the type of phosphodiesterase enzyme found in the blood vessels of the sponge-like corpora cavernosa running along either side of the shaft of the penis, which under the action of nitric oxide released by sexual stimulation becomes engorged with blood, producing an erection.

When he reported this interesting side effect to Pfizer head office in New York it caused quite a stir as the realization dawned that this magic molecule, nitric oxide, could potentially produce the highly profitable magic gun effect that men have always dreamed about. Well-designed controlled trials were rapidly set up, and it soon became apparent that Viagra was a winner in the erection stakes. It got surprisingly rapid licensing from the largely male Food and Drug Administration (FDA), who knew an urgently needed medicine when they saw one, and the rest is history.

Testosterone and Viagra – the dream team

While testosterone alone can restore full potency in about two thirds of men suffering from andropausal symptoms, and restore the libido in over 90 percent, this left a third whose minds were, as one patient put it, making appointments their bodies couldn't keep. While they could usually be helped by the methods described in the previous chapter, these were inconvenient and often only partly effective.

As soon as Viagra was approved by the FDA for use in America on March 27th, 1998, I got a US pharmacy to send me supplies for use on a 'named patient only' basis, which UK doctors can do with medicine not yet released in this country. The results were so spectacular, that I and the patients who were the first to try it were delighted and most impressed with its effectiveness.

The obvious thing to do was to see how effective the combination was of testosterone plus Viagra. I therefore contacted 100 patients who had failed to fully regain their erections on testosterone alone, and with their enthusiastic consent started them on Viagra, in addition to their usual hormonal treatment. Having read the initial reports on the safety and effectiveness of Viagra which had been published over the previous two years,[3] I recommend that the safest way to start is to use the smallest dose which gives a satisfac-tory erection with only mild side-effects. This means increasing the dose from 25mg to 50mg and if necessary to the full 100mg pill.

As absorption is slowed by food, it should preferably be taken 1–2 hours before sex for maximum effectiveness. Men who wanted a quicker action could chew the tablet and it would be more rapidly absorbed, but taste very bitter. This is why Pfizer is working on a new wafer thin lozenge which would be faster acting than the diamond shaped blue pill which most men instantly identify as Viagra.

The results were really impressive with this combined treatment, as I reported at a conference in America that fall[6], and at the WHO sponsored Second World Congress on the Aging Male held in Geneva in February, 2000.[7] The patients gave it rave reviews. Words like fantastic, marvellous, and magic were the most commonly used. In these first 100 patients, aged 36–81, it restored full potency in over 95 percent, and in a similar number it restored libido. While Viagra isn't supposed to affect libido, in these cases the added confidence it gave them knowing their erections were 'sure-fire' certainly seemed to boost their enthusiasm for sex.

In my study, the dose of Viagra judged by the patients to give optimal results was 25mg or less in 36 percent, 50mg in 52 percent, and 100mg in 12 percent. These doses were much lower than those used in other studies using this medication alone.[3]

I found that overall the effectiveness of the Viagra treatment was rated as 'very good' in 72 percent, 'good' in 20 percent, moderate in 6 percent, slight in 0 percent and ineffective in only 2 percent. The side effects experienced were flushing in 19 percent, headaches in 9 percent, nausea in 1 percent and blue tinges to lights in 5 percent. The side effects were only slight, and no one stopped the treatment because of them. The higher than expected frequency of flushing may have been due to the generalized vasodilator action of testosterone.

Many patients also reported that the effects of a single dose of Viagra seemed to last longer, allowing them to get a natural erection more easily than they expected, for an average of over ten hours (range 3–48). The patients noticed an increase in the number of erections the following morning and greater ease of obtaining and maintaining an erection the following day even without a further dose.

Some also told me that Viagra seemed to 'clear the system' and improve the quality of their erections between treatments, perhaps by lessening performance anxiety. Once they were confident that they could have intercourse with the medication, they tended to feel more relaxed without it, and erectile dysfunction became less of an issue both for them and their partner. Premature ejaculation also seemed to be helped, partly because the men felt they could maintain their erection, and didn't have to hurry before it collapsed.

Men who were asked to rate the effects of the combined testosterone and Viagra treatment on restoring their erectile function, said they felt on average 19 years younger (range 0–30). A few felt that they had reached a peak unsurpassed previously in their lives because they were more skilled at pleasing their partners, more considerate, and no longer suffered premature ejaculation. The angle of the erection, which normally declines with age, also appeared to be restored in many cases.

The authors of previous trials had emphasised that sildenafil does not enhance libido, and is likely to be ineffective in its absence, which is one of the reasons for giving testosterone. However, this study suggests that greater confidence in being able to perform physically improves the desire to do so, i.e. strengthening the flesh fortifies the spirit.

Because testosterone treatment relieves the underlying cause of the whole range of andropause symptoms, including particularly loss of libido, as well as the fatigue, depression and irritability which makes satisfactory intercourse less likely, in many cases it is worth a clinical trial before giving Viagra. In a third of such cases, where the erection problems do not respond, a low dose of Viagra is highly likely to complete the cure. This is partly because of the effect of testosterone in boosting libido, and also because animal experiments suggest it increases the production of nitric oxide in the penis by the nitrurgic nerves.[8]

One of the major benefits of the new treatment is a new concern for men's health issues and ways of promoting the health of the aging male. Subjects such as erection problems, which were once taboo, can now be talked about with other men, with partners, and also with medical advisors, which was often difficult BV, but is now much less so AV.

These results were confirmed in independent studies carried out in another London clinic by a colleague of mine, Dr Duncan Gould. Previously he had found that with erectile dysfunction in apparently nonandropausal patients with normal testosterone, and no other obvious cause for their problem, such as severe cardiovascular disease or prostate surgery, Viagra worked in over 95 percent of cases.[9] He then gave the drugs in the opposite order to andropausal patients, starting treatment with Viagra, and getting a good response rate in only 57 percent. When he added testosterone, he found that half of them didn't need Viagra.[10] Those who still did found that they could use a lower dose and only use it occasionally. This similarity of experience with the combined treatment makes us think that this is the way forward in treating ED associated with andropause.

There are now over 500 men in our combined clinic taking Viagra either regularly or occasionally when they feel in need of a boost. Sometimes it is just kept as a talisman in the bedside drawer, for use in emergencies. The proportion of mild side effects has stayed the same, or even decreased slightly because men get used to them or learn to manage on lower doses. There have been no serious complications in this group, even in those on it for the full three years since it first became available, some of whom have heart trouble or high blood pressure. Use of anti-anginal medicines or recreational drugs such as poppers containing nitrates remain the only contraindications to what is, in my experience, and that of many other doctors world-wide, a very safe form of treatment for a very common and distressing condition.

Safety issues

With Viagra having been in use for over three years, with more than 25 million prescriptions being written for over ten million men worldwide according to the latest figures, overall there is steadily increasing confidence among medical authorities in its safety. Approved by the

FDA in the US in March 1998, and by the European Medicines Evaluation Agency in September of that year, the medicine has now been passed by regulatory authorities in over 100 countries around the world. More than 300 million pills later, the medical and business news is still good.

This is in spite of a few scare stories in the newspapers by sensation seekers, about sudden deaths in men who happened to be taking Viagra, although none have been soundly based on scientific research.

For example, there have been scattered reports of a few sudden coronary deaths in elderly men on the drug. This is hardly surprising as heart disease is what I called in a book back in 1974 'The Western Way Of Death,'[11] and the underlying furring up affects blood vessels all over the body, including the penis. This is one of many factors causing erection problems over the age of fifty, and Viagra may tempt many aging men to try unaccustomed feats of sexual activity, even after a 'layoff' of several years.

This 'Death on Tummy' as it is called in Japan, is particularly likely to happen when the sexual partner is not the usual one. In some parts of the States, and doubtless elsewhere in the world, brothels offer clients who may even be in their seventies or eighties, a Viagra and tonic to brace themselves for the event. Usually, in this situation, there is little or no medical supervision. Also, because of their natural anxiety about their performance, clients are encouraged to go straight for the big one, and take the largest 100mg Viagra pill, rather than starting with 25mg and working up as safety considerations would suggest.

The medical safety data reported when this drug is properly prescribed and used is much more reassuring. There have now been more than 36 double blind placebo controlled trials, including 4,500 men taking Viagra and over 3,000 men taking a placebo. These trials involved men of different ages, backgrounds and states of health, including men having previous heart trouble.

Some of the latest and most reassuring evidence from the cardiovascular point of view is a report in the British Medical Journal from March 2001, from the independent Drug Safety Research unit in the UK.[12] This group looked at short-term events in 5,000 men receiving Viagra for the first time. The majority were in the 50–69 age group. Compared to the general population, there were 30 percent fewer than the expected number of deaths from heart disease in the Viagra group, and no cases of heart attack, stroke or death in the first month.

Although one can never entirely rule out long-term side effects with such a literally potent drug as Viagra, the specificity of its action in dilating the blood vessels in the penis, largely to the exclusion of others all around the body, is likely to make it a uniquely safe pharmaceutical triumph.

Other oral preparations

Following the Viagra breakthrough, other oral preparations are hard on its heels. Pfizer itself is working on more rapidly absorbed versions, which can be taken as thin wafers, or even as a nasal inhaler.

Bayer is testing a closely related product to Viagra, called vardenafil, and hopes to market it by the end of 2002. The advantage claimed for this drug is that it is much more selective for the type of phosphodiesterase found in the penis, PDE5. If this is confirmed, it will not only avoid the few Viagra side effects such as hot flashes, headaches, and blue vision, but will make it safe for people using nitrate vasodilators for angina. This will extend its use to people who could only take low doses because of side effects, and make it available to a wider range of patients. Similar claims are made for Cialis, a direct rival from Eli Lilly, due to be released about the same time.

Abbott Laboratories and Eli Lilly are releasing another oral drug, with a totally different action called Uprima (apomorphine hydrochloride). Taken under the tongue, it has the advantage of acting within fifteen minutes, which can shorten foreplay, and result in less disappointment when either partner changes their mind in the hour it takes Viagra to act. It works on the hypothalamic region at the base of the brain, stimulating the dopamine receptors in centers which promote erections.

Clinical trials in nearly 5,000 patients have shown it to be safe and to have an acceptable level of side effects, which mainly consist of nausea and headache, both occurring in about 7 percent of patients, and dizziness in another 4 percent. However, the success rate in producing erections was not as high as with Viagra, and it remains to be seen how the side effect to benefit ratio works out in routine clinical practice, particularly when taken together with testosterone.

Sexual life after Viagra

Having reported the remarkable medical upside of Viagra, some attempt must be made to predict the likely social impact of this revolutionary drug, to look at possible downsides, and to make a cost benefit analysis.

Can and will health care systems in America, Europe and Australia afford to supply Viagra or will it become an over-the-counter drug available in machines alongside condoms? So far, the general view adopted world-wide by medical funding agencies is that other than for patients suffering from a limited range of conditions well known to cause impotence, such as prostate operations and diabetes, this is a 'lifestyle' drug and should be obtained by private prescription.

This raises questions about how much of an effect on personal and family life a disability such as erection problems has to have before its treatment becomes a medical necessity to be covered by insurance companies or the state? To one man, experiencing a problem once a week might slightly reduce overall enjoyment of his sex life, while for another it might wreck his marriage. Another might be a young pornographic movie star, who might lose his job if he can't perform for hours a day. Yet another might be a homosexual who wants to 'pull a train' and can't. Which of these is a case for subsidized treatment, and where are the dividing lines?

What about the social effects of making intercourse possible by producing an erection in a drunken man who would otherwise be incapable, or in any homosexual or even heterosexual man who might become more promiscuous and likely to spread the AIDS virus? Who is to judge?

Women are also ambivalent about the effects of Viagra. Some greatly appreciate the improved quality of the sexual experience which they can have with their partners. Others feel that it was never that great anyway and that they have reached an age when they would rather forget about sex. Within six months of its launch in the US, the papers reported, 'Sex drug turns aged tycoon into errant stud,' and lawyers who were said to be considering the action against Pfizer claimed, 'The makers of Viagra should be liable for something like this. It's like giving a loaded gun to someone who has not been trained to shoot.'

This is certainly not the case in my practice where wives often feel that the drug has saved their marriage and restored a relationship where full sex can play its natural, important part. A few report that they feel less feminine when their partners use Viagra, because it's not just their sexual attractiveness turning them on. However, because it is a more natural erection which comes on with sexual excitement, and goes down after ejaculation, it would seem the most natural aid to relaxed sex between loving partners. This is certainly preferable to methods where the man has to go off to the bathroom to jab a needle in his penis or put it in a vacuum device to achieve an erection.

However, such benefits haven't stopped the actress Zsa Zsa Gabor from recently filing a suit against Pfizer in the US courts claiming that her husband had become a Viagra addict, and after some years of usage couldn't make love to her without it. It will be interesting to see whether her complaint is upheld, as it seems to ignore the effects of advancing years on both of them. Although Viagra, particularly when combined with testosterone, can slow the march of time in relation to male sexual performance, or in some cases even reverse it by several years, it cannot be expected to stop it altogether.

This brings up the interesting question of its long-term effects on patterns of male and female sexual activity – how much will it affect marriage and other long-term relationships? Should Pfizer be forced to issue a health warning on the side of the packages saying 'This drug can seriously affect your marriage?' Time and popular opinion alone will answer these questions, but so far the practical benefits seem to far outweigh these theoretical dangers, and the magic gun shows no sign of backfiring.

Financial performance

A crude but effective measure of the impact of any major new drug on the medical market is how well the shares of the company producing it fare over the succeeding years. In this case, according to the latest performance figures for Pfizer over the five years to the end of 2000, share prices have increased by nearly a factor of five. This is well above either the general pattern of stock market prices, which until the crash of early 2001 had about doubled, or a peer group of pharmaceutical shares which had tripled. The biggest surge in Pfizer shares coincided of course with the launch of Viagra in 1998, but has been generally well maintained since. This appears to be a big financial vote of confidence in the drug, with no sign yet of a medical downside affecting the company's fortunes. The sheer scale of the triumph of pharmacological science is amazing. Worldwide sales of Viagra have risen to well over one billion US dollars annually. It is now among the most widely prescribed medications in the world, with more than 45 million prescriptions having been written by more than 500,000 physicians for more than 15 million men. In 2001 Pfizer UK was even given one of the Queen's Awards for Innovation, a sure sign of an up and coming product. Also in 2001, Pfizer Canada was given the highest accolade within that country's pharmaceutical industry, the Prix Galien.

With Viagra, Pfizer claimed the big prize in this race to be first past the bedpost and help men with ED, but other closely related drugs are already under development. There are more glittering rewards for those who can copy or improve on this mighty feat of molecular engineering which made sure-fire erections possible for previously impotent men, the magic gun of their dreams.

Chapter nine

Secrets of vitality and virility

What conclusions can be drawn from these ideas about factors affecting men's health at different times of life? I believe there are lessons for society, as well as individuals living in that society, and what affects the well-being of one will affect the well-being of the other. Pollution of the external environment with xeno-estrogens for example, can have lifelong effects on the male, from causing the birth of a child with impaired sexuality to creating a subfertile male more prone to having a severe mid-life crisis and premature andropause. Probably the best way of drawing these strands together is to consider the causes of andropause, the changes needed to avoid it and the way to treat this drop in both vitality and virility.

The male psyche under threat

The fight for masculinity is a lifelong battle, with both chemical and psychological warfare involved.

First, in order to produce a male infant best equipped to maintain his masculinity for life, we must identify the sources of xeno-estrogens in the environment and then reduce them. The 'battle of the sexes' could also be called the 'battle of the hormones,' because generally male and female hormones have opposite and opposing actions, and currently, men are losing the fight, as seen in the falling sperm count.

Many of the battlegrounds are social and psychological, so these also need to be considered when planning for the future health of men.

This struggle is evident in everything from clothing to work. For example, besides reducing fertility and testosterone levels by raising the temperature of the testes, jeans are also symbolic of the identity and role crisis in the adolescent male. If everyone is wearing the pants, mentally as well as physically, what's so special about being male?

Also, there is a trend for women to be more sexually assertive, both in the East and West. In Japan, a few of what used to be shy retiring office girls are flaunting their sexuality, dancing provocatively in the scantiest of costumes during *bodycon* (body consciousness) evenings, stuffing bills into the posing pouches of well built male strippers and choosing a string of lovers. In the West, the feminists, having gotten most people thoroughly confused about what is really expected of the 'New Man' are now tending to turn to each other, and there is a fashion to alternate between heterosexual and homosexual relationships. There are groups for women who want to experience dressing, walking and talking like a man. Meanwhile, some young girls are tasting the delights of gang warfare and forming bands of highly aggressive muggers who occasionally become killers.

Increasing numbers of men who used to bond through body contact activities such as the football field are now holding hands and exploring the feminine side of themselves in encounter groups.

Many men stagger away from the divorce courts with little more than the clothes they stand up in, while alimony, palimony and child support lessen their financial independence. Loss of work from factors such as computerization and the world-wide recession can also cast husbands in the unaccustomed role of househusband. This can make them feel redundant both socially and sexually. In the intellectually prestigious Oxford Union, women debate the motion, 'A woman needs a man like a fish needs a bicycle.'

In my practice I am seeing increasing numbers of young men in their teens and twenties with what could be called the 'locker room syndrome.' This is an anxiety state where they do not feel sufficiently masculine in terms of their physique, body hair or penile proportions. In its fully developed state it can cause agonizing self-doubt to the extent that they avoid sexual relationships altogether, stop playing team sports which might involve communal bathing afterwards and in extreme cases even avoid public urinals where infavorable comparisons might be made.

This is made worse by the increasing sexual experience of women. They may have had several better endowed lovers in the past, or they have seen hard or soft-porn videos or magazines. These, as the young men are painfully aware, always feature handsome, muscular males well equipped to have sex nonstop. As one Indian Army officer said after watching a mammoth performance by a male elephant in 'must' servicing a female, *'That's a tough act to follow.'*

This is a difficult condition to treat and endless reassurance along the lines of *'It's not the size that counts,'* doesn't seem to help. General psychosexual counseling, sometimes over several months, together with assertiveness training, and hopefully a loving supportive relationship with a partner, gives the best hope of a cure. Sometimes a brief course of testosterone in low doses can produce more assertiveness, boost confidence and induce a more macho mood in which the penis seems more adequate and erections are stronger. Penile extension operations, even in men who are in stable relationships and have fathered children, are beginning to be performed on National Health Service patients in Britain and in private plastic surgery clinics throughout the world. However, an operation may well not be successful and this seems an expensive physical approach to what is essentially a psychological problem.

Other factors are also making women, particularly in mid-life, sometimes feel sexier and act more assertively than their male counterparts. Just as increasing numbers of businessmen are fading fast due to an unrecognized and untreated andropause, many women are coming into their managerial prime. Both in business and in bed men feel they can't keep up with them.

Does this mean that businessmen are now beginning to feel sexually harassed? In America increasing numbers of men claim to be, and lawyers specializing in this new crime are thriving. There is interesting research finding that more confident and dominant women show higher levels of testosterone than less assertive, stay at home types.

With all this pressure on men, no wonder the male mid-life crisis is striking with increasing frequency and severity. Suicide rates in men, always more frequent than in women, are increasing rapidly. A recent study in Britain by the Samaritans organization called *Behind the Mask* showed that over the last 15 years women's suicide rates had halved, while men are four times as likely to take their own lives, especially between the ages of 35 and 44, the peak mid-life crisis years.

Apart from their higher suicide rates, more men die from accidents at all ages, particularly when young, from car accident injuries. Also, although women generally complain more about their health, the number of life-threatening illnesses they suffer is generally less than the male, and more is spent on their health care. In Britain, as most developed countries around the world, large amounts of money are spent on screening for cancers of the breast and cervix, which are decreasing, while men have virtually nothing spent on detecting prostatic or testicular cancers, which are becoming more common. However, in the USA and Canada in the last few years men have been getting more screening for prostate cancer and in these countries death rates from this 'silent killer' are beginning to fall.

As a result of these combined factors, the life expectancy of men in most Western countries, including the USA and UK, is seven to eight years less than that of women. Is this an unalterable fact of life or would better health care for men, including hormone replacement therapy with testosterone, narrow the gap? We should urgently be trying to find out.

One of the countries with the lowest gap in life expectancies is Greece. Greek men also have one of the lowest heart attack rates in Europe. Although this is doubtless due to the benefits attributed to a 'Mediterranean diet,' there would seem to be other psychological and cultural factors at work as well. It is worth looking to see what we might learn from their experience, without holding it up as ideal, desirable or even practical for most men.

In Greece the birth of a male child is a matter for great rejoicing, whereas the parents receive sympathy when a girl is born. Sons are the center of attention in the family, and are spoiled continuously and indulged by their mothers, sisters and grandmothers. At school the boys are outgoing and develop a wide circle of friends, which during adolescence form a supportive in group, or *parea*, who stand by each other loyally for the rest of their lives. Youthful depression and suicide are relatively rare, although car accidents, drugs and AIDS are taking an increasing toll. Marriage tends to be late and to a considerably younger woman, and according to the Greek Orthodox tradition, divorce is relatively rare. Partly this is due to having a well-worn escape route down to the local *cafeneon*, where a man can be comforted by his all male support group. For them it is better, cheaper and more fun than psychoanalysis.

Unlike the majority of British men, with their usual distant manner and stiff upper lip, physical contact and letting their feelings out is part of the way of life for Greek men at all ages. Both men and women sing, dance, laugh, weep, hug, kiss and literally pat each other on the back at every opportunity. As well as being in touch physically, they enjoy eloquent, spirited, emotionally charged conversations punctuated by laughter and decorated with gesture. Being cool, cut off and alone is thought to lead to loneliness, which is considered to be the worst of human afflictions, whereas good company, together with food and wine, is the elixir of life.

The Greek man often does more than one job, which tends to keep him active and employed to a respected and ripe old age. Late in life he is lovingly supported by his wife, sisters and daughters and daughters-in-law and generally cared for at home until he dies. This lifelong pattern keeps his testosterone and level of sexual activity high throughout.

A recent study of young Greek soldiers showed levels of testosterone at the upper limit of normal and very high rates of sexual activity, with one ejaculation per day on average. This seemed to be proportional to the amount of dihydrotestosterone (DHT), one of the breakdown products of testosterone, rather than testosterone itself. However this may have been a result rather than a cause of their vigorous sex lives and doesn't agree with other evidence that suggests that testosterone itself is more important in regulating libido.

At the other end of the scale you have the former Greek Prime Minister, with the appropriate doubly, if not trebly, androgenic name of Andrea Papandreou, who in his eighties scandalized his nation by marrying an airline stewardess in her twenties.

This does not mean that I recommend such drastic remedies to my patients or that such idyllic female support as Greek men traditionally enjoy is widely available in most men's lives, but I do think that there are important lessons to be learned from Greek male life patterns, and you will hear them echoed throughout this discussion on how to retain vitality and virility.

The flight plan for life

Life can be compared to a trip in a glider when, after being catapulted in our teens and early twenties to the peak of our innate physical and mental abilities by a powerful cocktail of hormones, including particularly testosterone and estrogen, we then go into a variable glide path for the rest of our lives, the rate of descent largely being controlled by the body's hormonal balance.

As already explained, some hormones, particularly the stress hormones such as adrenaline, noradrenaline and cortisol, increase wear and tear and the rate at which we use up our energy, having what is known as a catabolic (or breakdown) action. Others, particularly testosterone and estrogen, have the opposite, or what is called anabolic (or build-up) effect. This can explain why some people burn themselves out and go into a nose dive, their health crashing at the age of 50 or earlier, while others glide gently on into their 80s or even 100.[1]

These aging processes affect particularly the heart and blood vessels and, in the form of heart attacks and strokes, are the number one killer of Westerners, as I described in *The Western Way of Death: Stress, tension and heart disease*. Coronary heart disease is also the main reason why, on average, the life expectancy of men in Western society is so much less than that of women.[2]

In general, both physically and mentally, you're as young as your arteries. So, as testosterone and estrogen have both been used to prevent and treat heart and circulatory disease, and also maintain the condition of the skin, muscles and bones, it seems reasonable to expect that we could use them to slow down the aging processes and prolong active and enjoyable life.

Age, stress, alcohol and drugs are, as already discussed, the main factors in bringing on andropause, so any plan to maintain vitality and virility must take these into account. Although you can partly do this on your own with the help of this book, it is much better to have a medical adviser to guide you individually. At the risk, as elsewhere in this book, of offending the politically correct lobby, I would suggest this adviser should be male, and probably in his forties, fifties or sixties so that he has plenty of experience and knowledge of the problems, having successfully solved many of them himself. Ideally he should be one of that currently rare breed, the andrologist, with a broad range of graduate training and specialized interest in endocrinology as it applies to men, as well as knowledge of fertility, erectile and psychosexual problems. Alternatively, an experienced general practitioner who has read widely on the subject, particularly if he has attended courses on the more specialized areas of andrology, could be a good adviser. Perhaps most important of all is to find one you can confide in and relate to, and whose opinion you respect.

Whoever you choose, he should be able to tell whether you are going through a mid-life crisis or male menopause and to help you through both. In other words, by a review of your long-term health record, together with how you feel and how you function, and by a detailed medical screen as described in Chapter 6, you can find out which glide path you're on and what flight corrections are needed. Many of these corrections will be self-evident while others will need a more objective or detailed analysis by your medical adviser.

Slowing aging

A population peak of 'Baby Boomers' is now reaching the age of 50. This affluent group has generally more leisure and disposable income than earlier generations and is tending to retire earlier. They therefore have higher expectations for the quality of their lives from 50 onward and are unwilling to tolerate the symptoms of menopause. Already having wealth, they also want health and happiness to go with it in what should be the 'golden years.'

Health maintenance, or what used to be called preventive medicine, is a relatively undeveloped and unsuccessful science, at least as far as the middle and later years are concerned. Coronary prevention studies such as the Multiple Risk Factor Intervention Trial, mistermed MR FIT, have generally proved uniformly unsuccessful, any small reduction in heart disease being outweighed by increased deaths from accidental deaths and suicides.

Similarly, as an article in *The Times*, 'Behind the Screens,' pointed out, routine medical screens, although seeming like a good idea at the time, and taking up considerable private and public resources, have not in fact made any appreciable impact on either morbidity or mortality in any area, especially cancer. Indeed, as this thought provoking article emphasized, by causing needless expensive and anxiety provoking further tests, and causing investigation and treatment related disease, screening has so far done virtually nothing to either add years to life or life to years.

There are, however, some rays of hope on this otherwise gloomy scene. We need to look in some new directions. Here are some of the most promising.

Hormone replacement therapy

Slowing down the aging process is a combined operation. As already stated, you need to promote those activities which maintain, build up or restore mental and physical function, and reduce those which cause wear and tear and breakdown. While there is of course much more to aging than hormonal decline, I believe there is a strong case for promoting and prolonging a youthful balance of hormones by careful supplementation of the 'hormones of youth,' i.e. estrogens in women and testosterone in men.

The safety and effectiveness of carefully and cautiously applied testosterone treatment has already been described in detail. It shares many of the benefits of estrogen therapy, both in the treatment of symptoms of menopause and in all around mental and physical health maintenance. Both estrogen and testosterone can be regarded as anabolic or body building steroids.

If the women in a man's life is either younger than him in years or hormonally younger because of hormone replacement therapy, it seems to help to keep him young as well. This is provided the distance between the two is not so great that the bridge falls down.

'His and hers hormones' are certainly usually preferable to the other option of a man getting a divorce and marrying a much younger woman in order to regain his lost youth. Aside from the pain to the former spouse and the rest of the family, there is the emotional, social and financial stress caused to the man involved, the most painful part often being separation from his children. Although the new marriage may appear to be working for a year or two, as the divergence in interests and energy levels becomes more marked, the much older man is usually left trailing mentally, physically and, perhaps most importantly, sexually, and the relationship often falls apart with extreme unhappiness on both sides.

Attitude to aging is also important. With improved health care throughout life, especially with HRT, women are expecting to remain mentally and physically active, and to look and feel good for much longer. They see celebrities such as Joan Collins, Catherine Deneuve and Elizabeth Taylor looking as young and attractive in their fifties and sixties as they did in their forties, and have similar expectations for themselves. Increasingly men are having to think seriously about how they are going to keep up with their hormonally reactivated wives.

Some just give up and become couch potatoes, slumped inert in front of the television. Others try to rise to the occasion by going on a diet, giving up smoking and joining a gym or participating in more sports, but these efforts often fade rapidly, given the negative mood and inertia accompanying andropause. Maintaining a positive attitude is an important part of the 'flight plan for life' and this is greatly helped by testosterone treatment.

Stress management

Stress is one of the major factors contributing to andropause and, as already described, works against testosterone both by reducing its production and by releasing stress hormones such as adrenaline, noradrenaline and cortisol, which have a catabolic action. It is important, therefore, that as part of your flight plan you become aware of your 'stress payload' and how well or badly you are handling it.

This is not to suggest that you should become a stress-avoiding vegetable. Stress has had a bad press, but it can in fact be the spice of life and a certain amount is essential for our health.

The original definition of stress in engineering terms is: 'a force which when applied to a body sets up strains within it.' So stress can be seen as a very necessary force which powers our lives. It is related to pleasure, performance and productivity by an upside-down U-shaped curve, which varies from person to person. In just the right amounts, what could be called the 'workout' sector of the curve, the upper half of the left-hand part, stress makes us fizz and function at an optimal level.

Where the bad image of stress arises is when the amount increases to the point where we are pushed over the peak of the curve into the 'burn-out' sector on the right-hand side. We may then blow a mental fuse and have a nervous breakdown or slide into a depression, or a physical fuse and have a heart attack or develop a stomach ulcer.[3] Some people, notably certain politicians, can carry huge amounts of stress, while other, more sensitive souls, who are often creative and artistic, find high-stress situations difficult or impossible to cope with.

Stress is actually very addictive, a big turn on, and the common chemical pathway to pleasure is the stress hormone noradrenaline. This is released by what I call the 'six-C situations': competition, car driving, cigarette smoking, caffeine consumption, cold bracing conditions and copulation or other vigorous physical activity. This has been confirmed by blood samples taken in all these situations.[4] In my early days of stress research, my cardiologist friend Dr Peter Taggart and I found *Guinness Book of Records* levels of noradrenaline in the blood of racing drivers immediately after a race, especially where they did well, although it was difficult to catch up with them later to study the other situations mentioned.[5]

If you have too little stress or stimulation in your life, you find yourself at the 'rust-out' point at the bottom left-hand side of the curve. This is seen in the unemployed and in some people who have to retire earlier than they feel they should. Rust-out can be just as much a cause of 'distress' as burn-out, and may be one of the reasons why there is more social unrest and crime in times of recession, when the devil is making work for idle hands.

It is easier to tell when we are understimulated and bored than when we are overloaded with stress. We tend to overlook the early warning signs of excess stress, such as falling function and no fun in work and social life, anxiety and depression, poor sleep and migraine or tension headaches, hypertension, raised blood cholesterol, eczema, asthma and a variety of other psychosomatic ailments.

Avoiding burn-out

What can we do to reduce our chances of getting into this over-stressed, 'burn-out' state?

First, we can try 'stress reduction,' that is, how we can reduce unnecessary and unenjoyable forms of stress as far as possible. Some work related and family related stresses are unavoidable, but others just pile up unnoticed over time and can be weeded out when you think about them or write them down as a 'Stress Inventory.' Some are just due to trying to cram too many things into the day, so choices have to be made. Some are due to driven Type-A behavior patterns or 'hurry disease' as described by the cardiologist Dr Ray Rosenman in his book *Type-A Behavior and your Heart,* in which he gives Type-A drills to modify this harmful lifestyle.[6] The 'time management' skills taught in business school can come in useful here.

Avoiding people and situations which we recognize as being stressful to us can also be helpful. There is a certain kind of person who is a 'stress carrier,' like 'Typhoid Mary.' Although such people usually show no signs of being stressed themselves, they leave a trail of devastation behind them in the form of overstressed people. As one American admiral put it when asked how he coped with the stress of his job, '*I don't take it in – I dish it out!*'

How can you cope with these people? Sometimes you can avoid them like the plague they are and not be around when they visit. Others are just unavoidable, but you may be able to explain to them the way they make you feel and work out a way in which your contacts with them can become less stressful. A very good manual of survival strategies in this situation is *Nasty People: How to stop being hurt by them without becoming one of them* by Jay Carter.[7] Transactional Analysis skills as described in the books of the American psychologist Eric Byrne, especially *The Games People Play,*[8] can also help defuse and prevent tension arising from contact with stress carriers.

The car is also a great stress-generating machine, as my research into stress hormone levels in different situations showed. The racing drivers' noradrenaline had the effect of raising blood fat levels, particularly neutral fat or triglyceride, so that the blood plasma became opalescent and milky after the race.[9] We also found that even in everyday motoring, noradrenaline and adrenaline levels shot up in most drivers, snarled up in a traffic jam or fined for parking. As I described in *The Western Way of Death*, men particularly are very attached to their 'ego chariots,' and 'machismo machines.' You see reactions of rage in and around cars during bumper-to-bumper traffic that you seldom see in other situations.[10]

At work, pecking order equals parking order. It is worth considering whether you can let the bus or train take the strain for some of the trips or traveling to work, or let the cabby's coronaries take the strain for getting around town. Again, society has a part to play here in encouraging governments to improve public transport, limiting pollution of the external environment by exhaust fumes from the traffic that clogs our roads and of our internal environment from the stress-related fats which clog our arteries.

Accidents are another source of stress and rapid aging, very often related to Type-A behavior: stress, tranquilizer use, drinking and driving, both on the road, at work and in the home. You may have seen in friends or relations how much a serious accident can age a person. Careful and cautious driving is to be recommended in avoiding accelerated aging.

My research on the effects of major trauma showed very high levels of stress hormones and marked lowering of testosterone levels, which reached crisis point about a week after the accident and could cause delayed deaths at that time from multiple organ damage, especially to the heart and brain.[11] Some of these effects could be reduced by stress-blocking drugs such as the beta blockers. Many of my patients dated the sudden onset of their andropausal symptoms to an accident or major operation, particularly involving surgery of the heart or prostate gland, so the fewer the operations you have the better.

Among its other advantages, so-called 'keyhole surgery,' using endoscopic instruments, may help to minimize operative trauma, postoperative complications and immobility, thereby lessening the wear and tear associated with operations, especially in the elderly. Also by reducing osteoporosis, testosterone is likely to make the trauma of hip, and other fractures less likely.

Stone Age reactions to stress

We have essentially not changed in our mental and physical constitution for thousands of years. Modern Space Age man still has his Stone Age psychology, physiology, biochemistry and endocrinology. His hormonal responses to a stressful situation are still the same whether it's fighting a hostile takeover bid in the boardroom or a sabre-toothed tiger in the jungle. In either stressful situation the primitive fight-flight mechanism comes into action, and the body is put into a state of emergency by the autonomic or automatic nervous system and the associated hormones.

How does this happen? Adrenaline speeds up the heart and mobilizes sugar into the bloodstream, while noradrenaline produces arousal, and raises blood pressure and fat levels to pump these fuels into the muscles, giving extra energy for fighting or running away. At the same time that these breakdown, catabolic processes are being switched on, the build-up, anabolic processes linked with testosterone are being switched off, because this is a time to make war, not love.

The problem in modern times is that our instinctual reactions to stress have become inappropriate. Much as we might feel like it, when in danger, we can't scream and shout and run around.

Let's look at the various ways in which we can balance up our stress responses.

Exercise

Physical exercise is one of the best and most natural ways of getting our mental and physical reactions to stress back into balance again. After exercise, the mind calms down, the tension in the previously coiled springs of the muscles is reduced, and the sugars and fats mobilized into the bloodstream have been used up. In this state of rest, relaxation and restoration, testosterone levels rise again, as has been shown in many research studies on people exercising. If you overdo it, however, and the exercise itself is pushed to the point where it becomes stressful, testosterone levels fall, as was shown in marathon runners. So, train, don't strain, and remember, exercise doesn't have to hurt to do you good – quite the reverse. No pain means safer gain!

With this in mind, and because andropause is mainly a condition seen in men around the age of 50, exercise in this group should be designed according to the acronym SAFE. It stands for Safe, Acceptable, Fitness producing and Economic, and is fully described in the book *F/40: Fitness on Forty Minutes a Week* that Al Murray and I wrote together.[12] ... Here is the summary:

S – *Safety* is the essential requirement for exercise in this age group of men. It should ideally be vigorous but not violent, calming and not overcompetitive, and isotonic, or dynamic, rather than isometric, or static, which causes the blood pressure to rise too much. A good safety check is the pulse rate, which can be taken by feeling it at the wrist or using a pulse monitor. This should not rise above a safe level, which can be calculated according to your age, fitness and medical condition.

A – *Acceptability* is essential as it is no use having the best system of exercises in the world if you never use it. Find the form of exercise you find acceptable to you and use that. The right surroundings are important. If you don't feel like going to a gym or swimming pool, a personal fitness trainer in your home may be the answer, as well as providing the necessary motivation.

F – *Fitness* in terms of feeling and looking better, and achieving greater strength and mobility, together with the relief or prevention of andropausal symptoms, are some of the benefits of exercise. These can be especially marked during treatment with testosterone.

E – *Economy* both in terms of time and money is attractive to most people starting exercise. Two 20-minute periods of vigorous exercise each week, or three times that amount of light exercise, are sufficient for most men to maintain a reasonable level of fitness, control weight, raise testosterone levels and keep sexually active.

Having covered the basic principles of exercise to maintain vitality and virility, let's take specific examples:

- Walking – This, like cycling, is a much underestimated and underused form of exercise which can replace more stressful driving while improving fitness towards taking on more vigorous physical activity. To give maximum benefit it needs to be brisk enough to raise the pulse rate to over 100 beats per minute, at least in the unfit. This means really striding out, what I call 'power walking.' Twenty minutes of this daily will give a good level of fitness in most men over the age of 50.

- Golf can also be a good way to encourage walking in pleasant company, providing it does not become too competitive. Unless you find walking very difficult for any reason, beware the cart, which can spoil the exercise element in golf. Many patients find that testosterone treatment reduces their golf handicap, improves their concentration and strengthens their drive (*see Alan's story, pages 88–9*). Perhaps one day golf clubs will have to have special competition categories for those on or off anabolic steroids.

- Swimming is excellent total body exercise, especially for those trying to lose weight. It could be said that you get double the benefit with swimming, because you are not only burning off a lot of calories by exercising the main muscle masses of the body, but also using up even more in keeping warm because of the heat loss even in water at a comfortable temperature. Unlike land-based exercise, any excess weight is supported in the water and does not throw strain on the joints. It's also a sociable and enjoyable form of exercise, and the sight of a range of attractive women in revealing bathing suits may do wonders for the libido of the andropausal male.

- Exercising in the gym is becoming increasingly popular and some enlightened companies are even providing it in-house. Ten years ago, with Al Murray, I helped to establish a gym in the House of Commons to encourage Members of Parliament to be at least physically fit to govern, although it seems to still be seriously under-used. Favored exercises among politicians still seem to be horizontal jogging, running opponents down and leaping to conclusions.

- A good gym should include properly trained and experienced instructors who carry out an initial fitness assessment, including measurements of heart attack risk factors such as blood pressure, and keep a continuing watchful and encouraging eye on your progress. Exercise schedules should be tailor-made to the individual and progress carefully monitored in terms of 'perceived exertion,' i.e. how hard the exercise feels, as well as by pulse rate measurements.[13]

- Straining at heavy weights is to be avoided, as are push-ups. With push-ups you are lifting three-quarters of the body weight and this is too much like maximal isometric exercise. The blood pressure is greatly raised by this type of activity and because of the increased pressure in the chest, blood cannot get back to the heart.

Also avoid prolonged exposure to high temperature sauna baths after exercise. Research we carried out at Al Murray's City Gym in London and reported in the British Medical Journal[14] showed that at high temperatures large amounts of adrenaline are released, which can make the heart beat rapidly and erratically. This can be more unsafe than strenuous exercise, particularly in those with high blood pressure or heart trouble. Cold plunges after the sauna are also not a good idea, as we showed that they cause the release of noradrenaline, which produces a dramatic surge in blood pressure. All these violent circulatory gymnastics are best avoided if you are seriously interested in longevity.

Running and jogging

Unless you are already in training, running and jogging are generally too vigorous to take up immediately without a period of power walking for several weeks beforehand. Even then these forms of exercise have been accused of 'mass murder' by Dr Meyer Friedman, a leading American cardiologist, who would agree with the cautionary saying, *'The grim reaper also wears a tracksuit.'* One of his victims not too long ago was Jim Fix, the American running populist, who abruptly dropped dead in his tracks, and he also obviously had designs on several American Presidents, who tend to overdo the fitness kick. Carter had to be carted off from one run, Bush Senior was so bushed on another he collapsed and Clinton visibly declined every time he was seen jogging. They must have gotten confused at an early age about the literal and metaphorical meaning of Presidents needing to run for office. Either that or they are running scared of the 25th Amendment to the American Constitution, introduced after the cover-up of President Dwight Eisenhower's stroke in the 1950s, in which a President can be declared unfit to govern for health reasons.

Besides the dangers to the heart and circulation in running, in some cities there is an increasing chance of actually being run over. Getting mugged is another risk. Knee and ankle injuries are also common, and running on hard pavements has been shown to cause blood to appear in the urine from trauma to the kidneys. As with walking, well designed shoes with shock absorbent insoles are vital for both safety and comfort.

Mental exercise as an antidote to stress

While many doctors know about medication in relieving anxiety, few realize just how powerful a tool it can be in stress management. Lectures in medical school mainly tend to focus on the wonders of medication, giving a message which is reinforced throughout the medical career by bombardment with literature and free samples from the drug companies. There are so many drugs to regulate our mental state on the market now that you might be forgiven for wondering if any of them work effectively. Also, there are many worrying reports of side effects.

Stress related symptoms are actually trying to warn us of something and taking medication is often just like turning off the fire alarm because you don't like the noise of the bells. Many patients tell of a zombie-like, switched-off state they experience on tranquilizers.

Malcolm Lader, Professor of Psychopharmacology in the leading research center in the field, the Institute of Psychiatry in London, has reported on the severe habituation which comes with long-term tranquilizer use, their addictive properties and the acute withdrawal symptoms which occasionally occur with suddenly coming off them. He also created alarm and despondency among doctors and patients alike when he reported that CAT scans showed that long-term tranquilizer use caused shrinkage of the brain similar to that seen in alcoholics, apparently due to 'neuronal dropout.'

Given such information, many people would prefer to control the stress in their lives by meditation rather than medication. It can be very effective in the control of stress reactions, whether as one of the different types of yoga or in its modern Western forms.

Meditation is simply the direction of flow of attention, according to Patanjali, the eighth-century Indian sage who systematized yoga. Most of the time our attention is directed outwardly. This focuses it on all the different forms of stress in our lives. In susceptible people it creates a vicious circle of stress leading to increasing stress hormones and decreasing testosterone, which all cause symptoms which generate more stress and further unfavorable hormonal changes.

When attention is directed inwardly, which is what people usually understand by meditation, we become uncoupled from the stresses in our lives and the body's self-healing, restorative relaxation responses take over. This produces a switch from overactivity of the fight-flight 'war' system to increased activity of the rest-restore-relaxation 'peace' system, with corresponding hormonal benefits, including the restoration of testosterone levels.

Such voluntary control over the body's involuntary nervous system, the autopilot which regulates our responses to stress, is remarkably easy to achieve. There is a whole range of techniques to help, which originated with yoga methods in India, moved to China as Buddhist meditation and then to Japan as Zen meditation.[15]

Autogenic Training is a Westernized rediscovery of the basic principles of Eastern forms of meditation. Its essential basis is the sequence of the six standard exercises developed 60 years ago by Dr Johannes Schultz, a German psychiatrist working in Berlin, where an institute has been dedicated to his memory. Autogenic Training involves focusing the mind by silent repetition of 'verbal formulas' suggesting sensations of heaviness and warmth in the arms and legs, a calm regular heartbeat, easy natural breathing, abdominal warmth and cooling of the forehead.

Under medical supervision, these mental exercises are progressively introduced at individual or small group training sessions held once a week over an eight to ten-week period. The patients then practice them in a comfortable, stable, sitting position on the edge of a chair, in an armchair or lying flat on their backs. Whether at home, in the office or traveling, they can usually find an opportunity for a session of 'Autogenics.' Usually the recommended practice time is 10 to 15 minutes three or four times a day.

You don't have to be a burnt-out stress victim to benefit from Autogenic Training. It has been widely used in industry and, being noncompetitive and nonintrusive, can be taught on in-house courses. It has also been taught to airline pilots and has proved helpful in coping with jeg lag. It was one factor that the training of both astronauts and cosmonauts had in common. It has also been used extensively with competitive sportsmen and women, along with musicians and others in the performing arts. There are many fringe benefits, such as reducing the amount of sleep required and promoting creative thinking by balancing the two sides of the brain, the logical, linear-thinking left and the intuitive, creative right.[16]

For the andropausal patient, as well as reducing stress, Autogenic Training can help control alcohol and food intake gently but firmly over a period of weeks. The psychological effects can also help the person work out longstanding emotional problems both at home and at work. However, it must be emphasized that it is a practical skill, like learning to drive a car, and you need a well-trained instructor. Autogenic Training is relatively unknown outside Europe, but Britain is fortunate to have an organization called the British Autogenics Society (BAS), which can provide a list of trainers in most areas of the UK.[17] It is part of an organization called the International Committee for Autogenic Therapy, dedicated to making properly taught Autogenic Training available around the world.

Siddha meditation is the one Eastern technique of which I have practical experience and can warmly recommend as being a very simple and clear form of meditation. It is based on an ancient tradition and philosophies which help control and reduce strss, among its many other life-enhancing benefits.[18] It is a very spontaneous form of meditation, which is taught in over 600 centers all over the world, including North and South America, Britain and the rest of Europe, Australia and India, where it originated and is respected as a great tradition. There is a branch of the Siddha Yoga Foundation in most countries and a center in most major cities. The current head of this lineage of meditation teachers is a beautiful Indian teacher called Gurumayi Chidvilasananda, the successor to the revered Swami Muktananda.[19]

The technique basically involves calming the mind by focusing it on a simple word formula or mantra, linked with the breathing. This makes use of the age-old observation that when the mind is disturbed, the breathing is usually disturbed also. Conversely, controlling the breathing can help to control the mind. When the mind goes still, great feelings of peace and calm can arise from within, and subtly but powerfully change the person's life, as I and a number of my patients and friends have found.

Avoiding rust-out

Every person has an optimal level of stimulation or stress, and above and below it lies unhappiness. Once our basic survival needs are taken care of, as they increasingly are in most societies, and we have fulfilled our 'biological imperative' by having and bringing up our children, what do we do then?

There is an old saying that what you don't use you lose. This is true in terms of mental, physical and sexual function. You see it every day in people who retire, sink into apathy and often die soon afterward. It is also seen in younger people made redundant who give up hope and give up trying to get a new job. In this situation it is probably better to do anything than do nothing.

It is one of the tragedies of modern life that there seems to be polarization of the workforce. At one end you have the overemployed, who are risking burn-out by working longer and harder to keep their jobs in the face of seemingly ever increasing competition, and at the other you have the growing ranks of the rust-outs who are unemployed or have been forced into early retirement by rationalization and down-sizing of their firms. Both groups can be equally unhappy, but for opposite reasons.

The Protestant work ethic isn't working any longer either, because it is increasingly absent for a large number of people for a large part of their lives. During the twentieth century more and more people have moved into urban environments, with a corresponding reduction in manual work. The proportion working in agriculture has fallen in America from about 20 percent to 2 percent. The 9–5 till 65 is no longer even the structure of the city dweller's life any more. What's to take its place?

Beer and circuses were the answer during the decline and fall of the Roman empire, and perhaps beer, game shows and the rest of pulp TV are the modern equivalent. Yet beer, combining the hazards of both alcohol and phytoestrogens, certainly doesn't do much for either vitality or virility, and TV mainly promotes endless unsatisfying consumerism and discontent. What are the alternatives?

It is surprising how little either politicians or sociologists appear to be looking into this question, since it seems that one of the main problems to be faced during this millennium is that work as we know it today is set to become a luxury item. Perhaps occupation should become our preoccupation. Here are some suggestions to fuel the debate, since they have a bearing on how we face up to both the male mid-life crisis and andropause. A man without a function, after all, often ceases to function as a man.

Alternatives to work

Perhaps some of the answers to the problems being created by technology may lie in the applications of technology. For some people loss of a job has meant that they can discover new skills and abilities. They may find a new lease of creative life through the computer and even take to surfing on the Internet.

Others are seeking a low-tech answer and welcome the increased time available to them for pure recreation or self-development in a variety of ways. Some take to the worship of the small spherical object known as the golf ball, playing two rounds a day every day the weather allows them to. Some take up the search for spiritual enlightenment, and enjoy the structured life and discipline that either a church or yoga and meditation can provide them. Perhaps we need counseling centers to help people find their individual answers, or maybe even your friendly neighborhood andrologist could give some guidance.

Work sharing

As the number of hours of work needed to perform various jobs falls due to automation and computerization, so the need to share this now precious commodity increases. The trend towards teleworking makes such sharing potentially easier and more attractive in some areas. This can open up a new career working from home via modems, faxes and video-conferencing, without the expenditure of time, energy and money involved in commuting.

Imagine a system where the norm was a 16-hour working week, either two eight-hour days or preferably four four-hour shifts. If you were a morning person, you could jump out of bed and work in the morning. An evening person could surface more gently and work in the afternoons. Moonlighting workaholics would be gently weaned off their addiction in work withdrawal programs, led by teams of easy-going idlers. They would be reminded that the working day of the caveman was only three or four hours long and the rest of the time was spent in social activities such as tribal dancing or personal grooming before an evening around the campfire.

Work shortening

Not only might the working week be shortened, but the years worked might be shortened to 30 or even 20. The Brahmin ideal of life in India has four approximately 20-year periods: student, householder, progressive detachment and ultimate contentment. Having finished your education around the age of 20, you would then have the privilege of working for 20 years to establish your position in a less competitive society, to bring up your family, if you decided you wanted one, and to have some extra consumer goodies above the guaranteed social norm.

After your 20 years' work, the mid-life crisis would be much less of a problem, because it would be expected that you would take up some more creative or leisurely pastime or study. Rather than 'retiring,' you would be advancing in some new direction and might wish to take a few years to attend a 'University of Mid-life' as a mature student to go deeper into something that you might have missed out on previously.

This period of detachment could also lead to more unpaid volunteer work in the community, and perhaps be a time for some to do more social work or counseling. Some could even take up political pursuits, using their life experience and maturity, which would be greater than the average career politician. It may be, however, by this time that the person will have come to the same conclusion as the philosopher who set out as a young man to change the world, and with increasing experience progressively narrowed his activity to changing his community, to changing his family and friends, to finally just trying to change himself.

Work shifting

There are some jobs, mainly in the so-called service industries, that just can't be automated. These range from psychotherapy to hairdressing, i.e. sorting out the inside and outside of the head, and from medicine to massage, i.e. making the inside and outside of the body feel better. Shifting work into these often overstretched professions would create many new satisfying jobs, and could well improve the sum of human health and happiness.

For those who wished a more action-packed time in their lives, short periods of volunteer overseas service in teaching survival skills or bringing aid to developing countries or disaster-stricken areas might provide the ideal opportunity.

Power sharing

A study of the health of London civil servants, the Whitehall Study, which has been going on for about 30 years, has shown that those in senior positions, the 'mandarins,' enjoy better health and tend to live longer than those in the middle or lower echelons. Perhaps the answer to this interesting observation lies in the original meaning of the word 'mandarin,' which was 'a high civil servant thought to exercise wide undefined powers outside political control.' The power element may well be linked to testosterone levels, because, as we have seen, the sense of power promotes secretion of this hormone. This is seen throughout the animal kingdom, but particularly in aging stags, bull seals and male primates.

Taking this idea a step further, sharing power and empowering people in different areas of their lives could well help to maintain their hormone levels. This would range from setting up managerial structures with a broader power base to setting up production lines, as in the Volvo experiment in Sweden, where one worker sees his product through from one end to the other, rather than performing only one limited task. Similarly, the American telecommunications company AT&T has extended the powers of an increasing number of their operatives to follow up and provide a larger range of services to the customer who first contacts them and becomes 'their client.'

The rapid improvement in communications may also empower people by letting them take part in decision-making processes at both a local and national level. Via telephone and fiber-optic links they could make their views felt in polls and referenda, and even add a new dimension to the deliberations of their governments by voting live on issues which concern them, making democracy a more exciting, interactive process.

Alcohol

Alcohol is one of the major factors contributing to male menopause, and if there is a serious alcohol problem it is not worth giving testosterone until it has been treated with the help of one of the effective agencies such as Alcoholics Anonymous. Also, as already described, the testis is very sensitive to both the short and long-term effects of alcohol, even in amounts which are insufficient to damage the liver or cause social problems.

Also, because of the phyto-estrogens in beer, which may still be present even in low alcohol types, it seems worth trading the beer intake for wine, especially red wine.

Diet

Weight reduction is often needed to help in the treatment of andropausal symptoms. In fact weight gain which doesn't respond to diet is one of the most common and demoralizing effects of this condition. Often this is mainly in the lower abdomen, giving a 'beer belly.' One witty journalist said that until the age of 40 he used to be proud of the breadth of his mind and the narrowness of his waist. Then he woke up one morning and found they had changed places.

The spreading waistline is a sign of andropause and makes it more severe. This female type of fat distribution is partly due to the action of the estrogenic factors which may have helped to produce it in the first place and partly because when there is more fat in the body, resistance to the action of testosterone increases and more of it is converted to estrogen. Testosterone deficiency also causes more sugar and protein to be converted to fat, so there is a general tendency to put on weight. As the couch potato grows, energy decreases, less exercise is taken and, lacking both activity and testosterone drive to build them up, the abdominal muscles melt away as the paunch appears.

Fortunately, as well as restoring the will power, or rather the won't power, needed for successful dieting, TRT improves sugar metabolism so that less is converted to fat and more goes to rebuilding the muscles. The effectiveness of this form of treatment was shown in a study in Göteborg in Sweden, where the cosmetic effect in reducing beer bellies, as well as the other benefits of testosterone treatment, was greatly appreciated by both the patients and their partners.

As with alcohol-related problems, expert guidance in specialized groups such as Weight Watchers or in the many health clinics specializing in this area may be needed to help the patient really tackle his weight problem, especially after many years of inertia. Where there is marked obesity, this can be a very important factor contributing to resistance to the action of testosterone, essentially similar to the insulin resistance seen in adult onset diabetes.

On a related topic, psychopharmacology is making rapid advances in the field of so-called 'smart drugs' which claim to slow mental aging and the loss of memory which goes with it. These widely discussed but little applied drugs, combined with psychotherapeutic mental exercises and relaxation techniques, and the benefits of HRT in both sexes on cerebral function and circulation, should have enormous potential in 'brain maintenance.'

Various dietary supplements are on the market, which are claimed to increase libido and help avoid prostate problems. In particular there is an interesting Swiss Oat preparation which is supposed to free up testosterone by reducing the inhibitory SHBG. This may be one of the natural plant hormones which will find a place in the treatment of patients who want to avoid long-term orthodox hormone treatments.

Antioxidants and micronutrients

Antioxidants, especially Vitamins A, C and E, together with micronutrients such as selenium and zinc, are now widely discussed and taken, both to improve vitality and potency and to reduce heart disease and cancer. However, this is largely on a haphazard basis, without any medical authority or guidance.

I think there is now compelling evidence that vitamin supplements may have a generally beneficial effect in maintaining health and may well reduce heart disease in the long term. These effects may well be due specifically to their antioxidant effect, perhaps by reducing the so-called 'free radicals' which are supposed to contribute to these conditions.

Zinc is concentrated by the prostate gland, and is an important ingredient of the seminal vesicle fluid which joins the semen as it is pumped through the ejaculatory ducts in the prostate gland. Its function seems to be to activate the sperm, which appears to pump zinc just as the muscles pump iron. Like the vitamins, in sensible amounts it appears nontoxic and may be beneficial.

Men's lib

What I am advocating is boosting the vitality, strength and longevity of men of all ages, but particularly past the age of 50, to the point where it equals that of women, especially when the latter are on HRT.

This is a physical and mental balancing act to maximize the many benefits of testosterone in men. In no way does this mean testosterone for all, rather giving male HRT only when needed to treat male menopause or for long-term health maintenance in older men who choose that option. Generally it involves maintaining the body's natural supply of testosterone, seeing that, like the man, it remains free and active, and that its actions are not blocked by factors such as SHBG, estrogens or stress.

Men are about 30 years behind women when it comes to HRT for the wide variety of historical, medical and marketing reasons already mentioned. Hopefully they will not catch up rapidly as male menopause is more widely recognized to be a real condition which can and should be treated, and as the safety, effectiveness and many benefits to physical and mental health of TRT become recognized. I have tried to spell out clearly the primary importance of testosterone in maintaining vitality as well as virility, but we need more doctors and therapists with a special interest in men's health issues, willing to act as leaders in the fight for what could be called men's lib.

This is not an antifeminist movement, but a way of recognizing the need to empower men and help them to remain active and equal partners throughout long and healthy lives. The 'women's lib' movement has helped women achieve social and hormonal emancipation, but the men are now lagging behind.

In America this has given rise to a men's movement which has psychotherapist Jed Diamond as one of the leaders. Diamond has written several important books on men's mid-life crisis and their menopause. On the psychological side, his writings on 'Getting back to the whole man,' in his books 'Male Menopause'[20] and 'The Warrior's Journey Home: Healing men, healing the planet,'[21] make a powerful case for men not living by testosterone alone, but also by developing a more mature form of masculinity.

In terms of longevity, women's greater life expectancy, when combined with the tendency for their menfolk to be on average three to five years older, according to actuarial statistics, means women lose their partners an average of 10 years or more before they die, which can make for a sad and lonely end to life.

It was the interest, enthusiasm and favorable experiences of the female public at large which brought in HRT with estrogens as a treatment for menopause. But the medical profession only belatedly woke up to the potential of HRT, as did the drug companies. May TRT receive quicker acknowledgement. Encouraging news on this front was provided by *The Times* of London on January 11th, 1996 when it was stated: '*The medical establishment now accepts that men, like women, undergo a menopause. HRT for men is on the way.*' The tide of public opinion is changing, as we will hear in the next two chapters.

It is my view that recognition of the reality and importance of male menopause, together with the present careful research of the rapidly expanding field of hormonal replacement therapy in both sexes, will lay the foundation for preventive medicine in the twenty-first century.

Chapter ten

Testosterone odyssey 2001

I would now like to give you a global view of the progress of the testosterone revolution in different parts of the world. Most of this is a personal view set against the background of over twenty-five years of traveling the globe talking to doctors, both in the academic field and in general practice, and to patients and their relatives.

An increasing amount of almost entirely favorable information is now available from the rapidly increasing number of published medical papers on testosterone and its effects, coming from researchers all over the world. So let's follow the ups and downs of testosterone treatment world-wide, as different countries have different stories to tell, and where you live may decide whether you can get male HRT easily or not.

United States

The favorable forties

Despite the work of pioneers such as Dr August Werner in St. Louis,[1] and Drs Heller and Myers[2] in Vancouver, Washington, D.C. and Detroit, throughout the 1940s in the recognition of and treatment of what was then called the 'male climacteric,' interest in the condition seemed to fade from sight shortly afterwards.

A book written in 1948[3] by Dr Elmer Sevringhaus, director of endocrine and nutritional clinics at the Gouverneur Hospital in New York, represented the peak of the forties enthusiasm for treating the 'male climacteric.'

This book, *The Management of the Climacteric*, gave a clear and logical account of the condition and its treatment as seen by the American pioneers in the field nearly half a century before, which coincided closely with my own experience. It quoted the previously reported view of the editor of the Journal of the American Medical Association that 'there is no longer clinical doubt of the existence of a male climacteric,' and recommended oral treatment with methyl testosterone, injections and pellet implants. The poisonous effects of methyl testosterone on the heart and liver, and its inexplicable continued availability in the USA to this day, is an important part of the remarkable twenty years of negative medical perception of testosterone treatment.

The writer and pathologist Paul de Kruif, whose book, 'The Male Hormone,' published in 1945,[4] did so much to popularize the idea of testosterone deficiency causing severe symptoms in men, unfortunately used this preparation himself. Through its unique adverse effects on the heart and liver, he may have succumbed to the long-term side-effects of methyl testosterone when he died in 1971, even though he was over 80 at the time. The thought that those who live by the chemical sword of testosterone might die from it, gives writers on the subject something to think about, if not 'meno-pause' itself.

However, in the last chapter of his book, having taken methyl testosterone for four years following the abrupt onset of his classic andropausal symptoms, he remarks that:

'Now I'm fifty-four years old, and there's so much left to do. I've grown old much too quick and smart much too late ... I feel that testosterone has already helped me. Of course the male hormone isn't the whole story. I'll watch my nutrition and go on supercharging myself with vitamins ... I'll stick to long hard walking in the dunes and along Lake Michigan in the wind and rain and sun. All this – plus methyl testosterone.

I'll be faithful and remember to take my twenty or thirty milligrams a day of testosterone. I'm not ashamed that it's no longer made to its old degree by my own aging body. It's chemical crutches. It's borrowed manhood. It's borrowed time. But, just the same, it's what makes bulls bulls. And, who knows, maybe tomorrow, they'll hit on a simple dietary chemical trick that will, to a degree, bring back the power of the glands that make my own natural male hormone.

Meanwhile I'll keep taking the methyl testosterone that now gives me the total vitality to go on working and waiting for such a not impossible discovery. Here's hoping.'

The nearest thing to the dietary supplement of his dreams to come along during the half century since he wrote so eloquently about the slow 'chemical castration of men,' is di-hydroepiandrosterone (DHEA). Although much used in the USA, probably because safe testosterone preparations are still limited there, it only raises testosterone a small amount. It may also boost estrogen production, adding to the harmful effects of these hormones in food and water, which can also contain other hormone disruptors such as anti-androgens, present in a wide and increasing variety of agrochemicals, preservatives, and plastic containers.

Overall, the environmental factors affecting men's hormonal balance may well have gotten worse rather than better since de Kruif's day, and testosterone antidotes are only just becoming more readily available again.

The dark ages of testosterone treatment

The years between the end of the 1940s and the beginning of the nineties could be called the dark ages of testosterone treatment.

As reported earlier in the book, this was largely due to the negative image of the hormone which developed in both medical and lay minds because of its abuse by athletes and body builders, as well as the prohibition by the Food and Drug Administration (FDA) in the USA of the safe and convenient medications which were allowed onto the market elsewhere in the world.

American physicians are only now taking more interest in the possibilities of male HRT and some excellent research work is being done at various centers in the USA on the uses of testosterone, particularly in diseases of the elderly. Let me tell you of the changing views which I have seen during my visits to the USA over the past twenty-five years.

When I visited cardiologist friends and physicians specializing in aviation medicine in San Francisco during the mid-seventies, interest in male menopause and testosterone treatment was approximately zero. While I launched into enthusiastic descriptions of Dr Jens Møller's work on treating impaired circulation in the legs with testosterone, which I had just witnessed at his Copenhagen clinic, they grew strangely silent and changed the subject. Lacking the scientific evidence to substantiate my enthusiasm, I learned to bite my tongue.

Even as an invited speaker on stress management at a conference held in Louisville, Kentucky, in 1979 during an International Symposium on Psychopharmacology, I could sense tension levels rising in the audience during a brief diversion into my talk into the effects of stress on hormone balance in general and testosterone in particular.

Not until 1987 was there a note of encouragement from a Professor Paul Rorch, chairman of the International Institute for Stress based in New York. As well as expressing serious interest in the part that stress could play in reducing testosterone levels and increasing resistance to its important actions, he was kind enough to send me a copy of the book by Sevringhaus[3] I mentioned before.

Again in 1991, while giving a talk on HRT for men at a medical center in La Jolla in California, I was met with extreme skepticism. Afterwards, while discussing whether the doctors there might consider setting up a clinic similar to the one I had in London, there seemed to me a marked lack of enthusiasm, and they treated me to a long lecture on the assumed lethal hazards of testosterone treatment. However this again was on the basis of their use of methyl testosterone.

By 1993, there were some signs that the climate of medical opinion was changing. Early in the year I was appointed Medical Director of a 'Hormonal Healthcare Center' in Honolulu, Hawaii, dedicated mainly to testosterone treatment for men. At the launch conference held just prior to its opening, we had several eminent speakers, including Dr Doug Soderdahl, a local American urologist, who appeared convinced of the need for testosterone treatment and of its safety in relation to the prostate, and hailed me as a pioneer. Dr Ronald Swerdloff from UCLA spoke of the benefits he had seen in treating osteoporosis in men with testosterone[5] and Dr Michael Hansen from Copenhagen spoke on its benefits to the heart and circulation.[6]

Unfortunately, some months after this promising start the clinic had to close because the only safe form of treatment available for routine use were shots of testosterone enanthate, which only lasted two weeks. Because of the general skepticism of local physicians and their unfounded fears about the safety of the treatment, they refused to send patients.

Meanwhile, a major media storm was brewing. A famous American writer, Gail Sheehy, who in 1991 had published a much acclaimed book on female menopause called 'The Silent Passage,'[7] did a detailed, but partly tongue in cheek, piece in *Vanity Fair* magazine[8] on 'Is there a male menopause?' This carefully researched article stirred up the academic hornet's nest surrounding the subject.

She had come to London to interview me and several of my patients at my Harley Street clinic, and had had glowing testimonials from them about the way in which testosterone had restored their vitality and virility, and found their experiences contrasted with the prevailing opinion among the majority of doctors in the USA at that time.

Part of the problem was that she mixed up the case histories of men experiencing the psychological effects of mid-life crisis with those caused by hormone deficiency in andropause. Also, she emphasized the erectile problems and lack of libido, which although common and important, are only part of the andropause problem, and until the advent of Viagra, the most difficult symptom to treat. Although hormonal insufficiency is generally agreed to be only one of several factors involved in erection problems, her article included 'expert' comments as extreme as 'A man does not need testosterone to have an erection.'

Her populist style and quotations from patients themselves who had been treated with testosterone, exposed her to a chorus of protest from American academics who said Sheehy's 'whole approach is a major problem.' Also they were quoted as hating to use the term male menopause and accused her of making it all up. Their view was that it was a mythical condition, and the rush to treat it would mean undeserved profits by unscrupulous doctors and drug companies. Some doctors were quoted as being openly hostile to my work.

Perhaps because of not wishing to risk future sales, when her article was partially reprinted as a key chapter in her next book, 'New Passages' a couple of years later,[9] a large part of the original version extensively quoting my work, had mysteriously disappeared – truly a bonfire of the vanities.

Dawn of the testosterone revolution

One long-term benefit of this very public controversy was that it prompted open-minded physicians in the field to at least consider that it might be worth exploring the symptoms caused by falling testosterone levels in men over the age of forty, and whether there could be any benefits for men with low levels of the hormone to restore these towards more youthful values. The National Institute for Health (NIH), one of the main grant-giving bodies in the USA, about the time of Sheehy's article asked for research proposals to investigate whether testosterone supplements might benefit older men by preventing bone loss, depression, and other symptoms associated with aging.

In 1994 a journal for American doctors called Hippocrates published a prophetic article in their 'On the Edge' series about new areas of debate in medicine. Called 'Hormone Replacement for Men,' it seemed to herald a shift to at least a more balanced consideration of the possibilities of this treatment. While it quoted opponents of the theory, it also mentioned those who were at least looking at the problem on its merits. After describing my views on equal opportunities in hormone treatments for the aging, the writer, Ingfei Chen, went on to say:

'Strip away the controversy, and what's underneath? So far only one fact has been confirmed within the last few years: As a man ages, his reservoir of active male hormone does drain away, although slowly. According to the Massachusetts Male Aging Study, a survey of 1,709 middle-aged men, blood levels of the "free" testosterone that interacts with the body's tissues normally subside at the rate of around one percent a year from age 40 on.

But does the smaller androgen stockpile matter? John McKinlay, an epidemiologist who coauthored the Massachusetts study says no. "I don't think there are any grounds for advocating testosterone therapy for aging men;" says McKinlay, who heads the New England Research Institutes in Watertown, Massachusetts. The Massachusetts survey found no signs of a "syndrome" resulting from so-called viropause, he and his colleagues say. Nor say the researchers, is there any evidence that changes in mood, energy, virility or fitness in older men are related to hormone fluxes.'

This large-scale, meticulously executed, multidisciplinary study, extensively funded by the NIH and other grant-giving bodies, started in 1987. Since then, it has been one of the main platforms for those opposed on theoretical grounds to the practical clinical experience of doctors and their patients that the typical pattern of symptoms of andropause could be relieved by testosterone treatment.

Only two years after it was set up, before the baseline readings had been completed or fully analysed, the authors cast doubt on 'The questionable physiologic and epidemiologic basis for a male climacteric syndrome'.[10] Summarily dismissing the clinical wisdom of two generations of doctors on the basis of a few preliminary observations from one incomplete study might be seen as a case of premature adjudication.

Indeed, there are now signs of a major shift in the study's conclusions as evidence accumulates that there are actually significantly low levels of testosterone in up to 40 percent of men over age 40.

Also, the study is now generating high quality scientific evidence that insufficient testosterone has adverse clinical effects in contributing to erection problems. In the same year it reported:

'Thus, diets low in protein in elderly men may lead to elevated SHBG levels and decreased testosterone bioactivity. The decrease in bioavailable testosterone can then result in declines in sexual function and muscle and red cell mass, and contribute to the loss of bone density.[11]

At the same time another article arising from the Massachusetts study looked at what might be taken as classic andropausal symptoms and concluded:

The importance of psychosocial risk factors should not be dismissed, however, and several cross-sectional studies have reported associations between ED and depression, anger, and dominance ... The results suggest that new cases of ED are much more likely to occur among men who exhibit a submissive personality.[12]

Meanwhile, back 'on the edge,' in the Hippocratic article of 1994, Ingfei Chen was able to quote two other American physicians who were taking a more positive view of the possible potential of male HRT.

> 'Other doctors at institutions such as Emory University in Atlanta, St. Louis University, and the University of California in Los Angeles, treat men over 60 for low testosterone reserves, but admit there's no solid proof of the therapy's benefits.
>
> In many cases, they say, restoring the hormone stockpile appears to improve strength and decrease body fat as well as vanquish mood and sex problems.'

Since then, the authorities she quoted in that article have had time to do some of the detailed studies which her article finished by saying were needed to make the case for the safety and effectiveness of HRT for men, and now take a definitely more favorable view.

Professor J. Lisa Tenover, who has established an internationally renowned geriatric unit at Emory University in Atlanta, has come from a point of healthy skepticism in the early nineties, to one of informed enthusiasm for the overall benefits of testosterone treatment in 2000. Showing kindness and support after the academic mauling I received at the First World Congress on the Aging Male in 1998, she explained at the Second World Congress two years later why her attitude is one of cautious optimism for the treatment.

When I visited her department in 2000, she showed me her very sprightly, and mentally alert older male patients exercising vigorously in the state of the art gymnasium facility there, and discussed the latest findings in her continuing research on male HRT.

> 'Reasons for this nascent enthusiasm include burgeoning evidence that testosterone levels decline with normal male aging (and with age-associated diseases) and an interest in preventing age-related dysfunction and prolonging quality life among an ever increasing population of older adults. The decline in testosterone with age often parallels unfavorable changes in organs upon which androgens act and the goal of male HRT would be to prevent, stabilize or even reverse some of these detrimental target-organ changes.'[13]

In the same year she is quoted as saying:

> 'When I first went into this area, I felt that what I would show was that, except for a select few men, it would be a bad idea. But the more I work with testosterone replacement, the less I feel that way.'

Also, she said that having reviewed the literature on this topic, although most studies have been small and relatively short, and gave testosterone by different routes, the findings were 'pretty consistent' in showing benefits for muscle mass, body composition, bone density and psychological status.

In start contrast to the very low official limit of 8nmol/l (230ng/dl) rigidly applied in Australia as reported later, because of uncertainty as to who will benefit, she is less stringent in treating patients in clinical practice than in enrolling subjects in trials. She is currently giving symptomatic men the benefit of the doubt, and offering them a therapeutic trial even though they may have total testosterones up to 14nmol/l (400ng/dl). She says she feels fully justified in doing so because

> 'I can double his level and still stay within the normal range. And maybe for him 400ng/ml is too low for optimal functioning.'

This view of an eminent and widely respected researcher is much needed encouragement for those of us who have been castigated for using similar guidelines for giving testosterone treatment for more than a decade, and catering for what we see as the needs of 'High-T' men.

Professor Tenover confirmed many of the benefits of 'Male HRT in the new millenium' as seen in her own placebo controlled studies, at the Second World Congress on the Aging Male in 2000.[14] She reported increases in bone mineral density, lean body mass, and improved mood and sense of well-being in the treated group. Even with the relatively high levels of testosterone reached by the injections she uses, there was no increase in benign or malignant enlargement of the prostate, or evidence of toxicity to the heart or liver.

These findings are entirely consistent with the mass of other recent evidence presented at the conference, which provided support for those involved in the therapeutic use of testosterone.

UK and Europe

The hostility and rejection experienced by Dr Jens Møller and Dr Tiberius Reiter to their work with testosterone in the 1950s, 60s and 70s has been described in Chapter 1. These were extreme examples of the attitude of the medical establishment world-wide at the time to male menopause and male HRT, and their work was studiously ignored and forgotten. However, in its usual circuitous fashion, medical opinion is swinging back to the acceptance and enthusiasm for these ideas which was briefly in vogue in the USA in the forties.

Much of the impetus for this change has come from Europe. In the eighties, when I started publicly supporting Møller's views that testosterone was positively good for the heart and circulation, there were howls of protest from national and international medical authorities who thought they knew better. Now to their surprise there is an avalanche of recent evidence that Møller was right all along, but unfortunately he didn't have full scientific information needed to prove his theories which were mainly based on careful clinical observation, to his highly skeptical critics.

However, Møller's loudly-voiced views probably acted like an irritant grain of sand which causes the oyster to form a pearl, and prompted some of the more open-minded physicians who he contacted and cajoled at meetings throughout Europe, to at least explore some of the radical ideas he expressed.

One of the most important of these was Professor Alex Vermeulen, working in the University of Ghent, who from the early 1970s to the present day, has done invaluable work on the decline in testosterone levels in aging males. Working with his colleague Dr Jean Kaufman, he has recently produced evidence confirming that it is the free active testosterone level which falls more from age 25 to 75 (50 percent) than the total testosterone (30 percent)[15,16] because of the increased binding protein in the blood. Using the current view that it is the drop in the man's present androgen levels compared to the high levels he had in his youth which determines whether he can be regarded as testosterone deficient, they found that more than 20 percent of men over 60 had low total, and a slightly higher percentage, low free levels of the hormone.

The most recent study by Dr Leifke, a German, looked at a large group of healthy non-obese men aged 20–80, who showed a mean lifetime fall of 51 percent for total testosterone, 64 percent for free testosterone, and 78 percent for bioavailable testosterone. These changes started in the third decade, and of the 60–80 age group, in relation to these different fractions of testosterone, 25 percent, 40 percent and 60 percent respectively could be considered androgen deficient by comparison with the lowest levels seen in the 20–29 age group.[17]

Professor Louis Gooren of the Free University Hospital in Amsterdam confirmed these falls, and completed a ten year study of oral testosterone treatment with Restandol, showing it was both effective and safe.[18] More recently, in a discussion of quality of life issues in the aging male, he raised the interesting question of why the halving of a man's youthful testosterone levels of 35 nmols per liter (1,000ng/dl) should be regarded as insufficient to bring on andropausal symptoms?[19]

This is an important question in relation to the seemingly high frequency of this condition if judged by the frequency of these symptoms in middle-aged and elderly men. If women can develop menopausal symptoms when their estrogen levels fall by half, why shouldn't men be expected to have similar symptoms when they have an equivalent drop?

Meanwhile, other German researchers, especially Professor Eberhard Nieschlag and his colleague at the Institute of Reproductive Medicine in Munster, Hermann Behre, have been producing further impressive and detailed evidence of the safety of even high doses of testosterone in relation to the heart and prostate, and defining the pharmacology and clinical uses of a wide variety of medications.[20]

The year 2000 was a turning point in the history of testosterone treatment for several reasons, as well as because of the evidence presented at the Second World Congress on the Aging Male held in Geneva in February, as described in the next chapter.

In March, my colleague in the London AndroScreen Center, Dr Duncan Gould, coauthored a paper in the *British Medical Journal* which helped greatly in turning the tide of medical opinion toward favoring recognition of andropause.[21]

This was regarded as so important for American physicians that it was reprinted in its entirety as Editors Choice in the prestigious Western Journal of Medicine in August 2000.[22]

The year ended with another important event, the launch conference of The Andropause Society (TAS) at The Royal Society of Medicine on December 6. This is a new web-based international charity which I helped to establish, with the aims of encouraging research, education and training about andropause and its treatment.

As far as we knew it was the first time an entire medical conference had been web-cast. Working with the established leaders in the field of broadcasting events over the internet, Camvista, from Kircaldy in Scotland, the society made the conference available to doctors world-wide, who could 'E-tend' from their home or office computers, live or any time later. This we believed was the next big step in medical video-conferencing techniques.

The speakers' talks and Power Point presentations, with high quality sound and images, were broadcast to the web. Doctors could then access just the sessions in which they were most interested, without wasting time in traveling and attending parts of the conference which were not relevant to them. This, the conference organizers predicted, is the shape of conferences to come, and is a major advance in medical knowledge management. The aim of this launch conference was to enable health professionals world-wide to hear the latest news, views and research of European experts in this rapidly expanding field of men's health. It made a highly successful conclusion to a key year in the history of testosterone treatment.

Canada

Since it was set up in 1998, the Canadian Andropause Society (CAS)S has become the leading organization of its type in the world. This is largely due to the initiative and drive of its organizing committee, especially the president, Professor Roland Tremblay of Laval University in Quebec.

Canada's dominance can be seen by the attendance figures for delegates from the various countries at the Second World Congress on the Aging Male 2000. Canada had 42 delegates, the equidistant but much more affluent and populous USA had 31 and nearby UK scored a modest 16, while Australia had just one.

An additional reason why Canada made such a good showing in this 'Andropause Olympics' was that from the outset its Andropause

Society has been well supported by the pharmaceutical company Organon. Although the company's headquarters are in Holland, it relies on the national subsidiaries in each country to market its products. As chance would have it, Organon had just launched its key oral testosterone product, Andriol (testosterone undecanoate), on the Canadian market. Along with sponsoring a web site for the society (www.andropause.com), it funded a most telling survey on the attitudes of doctors and the general population in Canada to the andropause concept.

This poll, organised by the Angus Reid organisation, was presented at the Second ISSAM conference by Dr McCready of Scarborough, Ontario, working with Organon Canada. The questions were put to a random sample of equal numbers of men and women, 1,500 in total, and 200 doctors. Analyzed separately, 70 percent of the lay group had heard of the term andropause, 80 percent believed it existed, and about half thought it could affect the quality of a man's life and might lead to more serious problems.

Of the doctors, 80 percent believed it existed, 70 percent thought that it could affect the quality of life, and 90 percent that low testosterone was a contributory factor. When asked what conditions might be related to low testosterone, other than sexual problems, 45 percent mentioned osteoporosis and 25 percent heart disease.

Overall, there was a surprisingly high degree of awareness in both groups of andropause and its effects, especially among women. With the usual attitude of high denial however, few men in either group thought the diagnosis might apply to them, although they could nearly all think of friends or patients it might. Most of the physicians were aware of the condition, but vague about its diagnosis and treatment.

On the basis of this survey, and the confident assessment of the national and international scene by the society, the home page of the CAS web site starts with the encouraging statement:

'The existence of Andropause is now recognized by the medical world – including the Canadian Andropause Society – and by Canadians alike.'

How has this victory in the world-wide testosterone revolution been won in Canada? As I saw when visiting Professor Tremblay in Quebec in the autumn of 2000, he encourages public awareness of andropause and its treatment by giving press and television interviews. He also tirelessly travels around Canada, as does Dr Alvaro Morales and several other members of his committee, attending and speaking at meetings of andrologists, endocrinologists and general physicians. This high level of activity in making the case for treatment of andropause not only inside, but also outside the medical profession, is now bearing fruit in seeing a high level of acceptance in both.

Combined with an ongoing research and teaching program, this makes the Canadian Andropause Society a model for organizations with similar goals around the world.[23]

Asia and the Pacific Area

From showing very limited interest and activity ten years ago, this whole area has become a hive of interest on the health of the older man and the potential for male HRT. As was made clear at the historic First Asian Meeting of the International Society for the Study of the Aging Male held in Kuala Lumpur, Malaysia in March 2001, the meeting focused very much on 'Managing aging populations – a global challenge.'

Typical of the many excellent papers from delegates from every country in the region was a message from the organizing chairman, Dr H. M. Tan:[24]

'In the developed countries, the percentage of the population of around 65 years of age will increase by more than 50 percent by the year 2025. The greatest rate of increase will be for the age group of above 80 years. With declining unsustainable birth rates, the traditional working population (age group 18–65 years) will face a huge burden if they have to fully support this aged population. Similarly, developing countries like China and Indonesia will experience the highest increase in the number of people above the age of 65 years. Their aged populations will more than double in size in the next 25 years. The sheer immensity of numbers will certainly strain the developing economies and their related social and political infrastructures.

Thus the problem of the aging poplation is universal, and in Asia where the majority of the countries are in the developing status, these problems may well be insurmountable if policy makers do not implement urgent and drastic steps well before this phenomenon occurs.'

This sense of urgency was also conveyed by other speakers from every part of Asia, and one got the sense that each was ripe and eager for the testosterone revolution to happen in their country.

Indonesia was facing the most severe problem with a forecast increase of over 414 percent in its aged population in the years 2,000–2025. Next came Kenya with 347 percent, Brazil 255 percent, China 220 percent, Japan 129 percent, compared to the relatively modest increases in developed countries such as Germany 66 percent and Sweden 33 percent. The contrast was stark and the thirst for knowledge on how to apply male HRT to maintain physical and mental activity, healthspan rather than just lifespan, was great.

While the knowledge of the nine invited speakers from the West was much sought and appreciated, there appeared to be less concern about the theory of testosterone treatment than the urgent need to apply it. Generally, while there was stronger support from the health authorities than is seen in most Western countries, who generally lack this sense of urgency, it fell to urologists to provide this form of HRT. The guidelines the Asian doctors recommended however closely followed the diagnostic and treatment criteria developed in the West.

Australia

Does male menopause exist in Australia?

Although I had been on lecture tours in Australia twice before in the seventies, talking at Australian Medical Association meetings and in university settings, giving papers to the attending doctors on stress, tension and heart disease, nothing prepared me for my next visit in April 1997.

I was warned to expect a macho culture, a nation of men in the mold of 'Crocodile Dundee,' all tough, virile, sporting, and dripping testosterone from every pore of their taut, muscular, bronzed bodies. Definitely the last thing they would need was advice on hormonal supplements from a whingeing pom. Also, there was the original title, 'The Male Menopause: Restoring Vitality and Virility,'[25] featuring a discouragingly droopy phallic peacock feather on the cover. For sure, no self-respecting Australian Male would be found dead clutching such a book for wimps. Only the cover of the book was hard.

Even though the Australian publishers tried to improve matters by printing the paperback version under the more upbeat title of 'Maximizing Manhood: Beating the Male Menopause,' the potential market for it did not seem very large. This view was reinforced before I even landed on Australian shores, when in the week leading up to my visit, the book was attacked on national TV by an Australian endocrinologist who described it as 'A mine of misinformation.'

However, his remarks and that of the interviewer made it clear that neither had read the book, as the points they raised had all been covered in it and referenced with published articles by leading medical experts. When challenged to a public debate, the equivalent of a 'testosterone test-match' on the same TV channel, he refused to be drawn.

When I finally arrived in Sydney however, the public response was overwhelming. My medical critic had only succeeded in stirring up a storm of media interest in the subject of male menopause and its treatment with testosterone. The resulting blaze of publicity was skillfully fueled by the public relations tiger organizing my tour, Linda Byart, whose energy and enthusiasm were and are, central to the ongoing struggle for male HRT in Australia. She is certainly one of the great fighters in the testosterone revolution as we shall see.

Linda was no stranger to the challenges of bringing about social change. Working with the British Safety Council for over 20 years, first as a senior executive and then as a consultant, she was responsible for campaigns that saved literally thousands of lives and prevented injury and damage to tens of thousands more. I first worked with her in the 70s and 80s while acting as a medical consultant to the UK British Safety Council campaigns on the effects of stress in the workplace.

After emigrating to Australia in 1988, Linda worked in public relations and marketing, and in 1995 set up a company in Perth specializing in performance enhancement and motivational training, personal development and public speaking skills. Her earlier battle training was very much needed in the fight for testosterone treatment in Australia which has continued and intensified since my first visit. Certainly, I have felt like a man who had sowed a storm and reaped a whirlwind.

From the first television interview in Sydney, the telephone lines at Linda's office were flooded with thousands of callers saying that they or their partners had the typical symptoms of male menopause, and asking where they could get treatment. This went on during dozens of national and local TV and radio interviews, both in Sydney and in Perth, and it rapidly became obvious that Australian men were as prone to developing the condition as those anywhere else in the world. Where were the doctors to cope with the testosterone related problems of so many men?

Fortunately, some of the respondents to the broadcasts and newspaper articles were doctors suffering from the condition themselves. First was a Sydney surgeon, who had just diagnosed the condition in himself, and after experiencing the benefits of oral treatment with Andriol, the local name for testosterone undecanoate (Restandol), rushed to my hotel to declare himself a convert, and asking to train with me.

The same thing happened in public and medical meetings in Perth, Fremantle and at the annual meeting of WACRARM (the Western Australian College for Rural and Remote Medicine). They came, they listened, their questions were answered, and they seemed convinced enough to want me to come back and train them in the skills of diagnosing and treating andropause. 'No probs,' as they say in Oz, or were there?

STAG at bay

Encouraged by the apparently huge unmet need for testosterone treatment in Australian men, and the enthusiasm of many of the doctors I had met to supply it, a second visit was arranged for me at the end of 1997 to train doctors in Sydney, Brisbane, Melbourne and Perth.

The person who made this possible again was Linda, who had used the 5,000 respondents to the previous publicity, including the doctors, to voluntarily set up a national organization called the Supplementary Testosterone Action Group (STAG). To raise awareness in the medical profession, and encourage more doctors to train, in November 1997 we set up an intercontinental ballistic medical event, the first medically accredited international video conference to be held in Australia.

In what we felt was an historic program, we had a live video link using the latest video-conferencing technology, despite the high cost of equipment and international telephone calls for a still embryonic organization hosting a program lasting several hours. Having stayed up most of the night in London installing the video equipment in my computer, it was a great relief that it worked.

It was a remarkable experience, and I and Dr Michael Hansen, a specialist in testosterone treatment of blood vessel disease visiting from Copenhagen, greatly enjoyed being able to talk face to face with about 100 colleagues on the other side of the world and answer their questions. We thought this would be the start of a 'Surfing Doctor Service' being added to the famous 'Flying Doctor Service' in Australia.

Encouraged by what was considered in both countries to be a successful event, I set off for what turned out to be a strenuous two week round Australia teaching tour. The tour which Linda organized on behalf of STAG covered teaching sessions to doctors in Sydney, Brisbane, Melbourne and Perth. Their enthusiasm, and that of the patients who had already started treatment, was both infectious and well, staggering.

The third tour was in August 1998, and was to help Linda and the growing number of STAG doctors set up 'Well Men' clinics and provide specialized facilities in most major cities in Australia. By then the 'Maximising Manhood' book was selling well throughout the country, and had even reached the best-seller list in Western Australia, so more doctors and patients had become interested in andropause.

One feature of all the tours was the sustained media interest in male menopause and the number of men contacting STAG to ask where they could get the treatment which they obviously urgently needed. Sometimes I got the feeling that Linda slightly overdid the rush to meet the long felt needs of the Aussie male. While I was still jet lagged and exhausted after a 20 hour flight from London to Perth, she kindly met me at the airport, and then took me straight into an interview and photo session with a major national newspaper.

One of the most supportive of the Australian doctors was Dr Adrian Zentner, a men's health and aviation doctor, who had been pivotal in setting up Well Men centers in both East Melbourne and Perth, and tirelessly traveled between the two, teaching, seeing patients and supporting Linda in her nationwide mission to further the cause of testosterone treatment.

One story he told from his extensive experience was of an airline pilot suffering the extreme fatigue which andropause can cause, who tried for no apparent reason to land his plane with several hundred passengers aboard on a major highway running parallel to the actual runway. When asked about this curious behavior, and what was in his mind while he was making this nearly fatal error, all he could say was that while coming in to land he was wondering why the runway had road signs on it.

This was one of many stories of the way in which lack of testosterone can ruin a man's performance both at work and at home. Human errors play a part in the majority of accidents, especially in aviation, as well as on the road and elsewhere and it is almost certain that andropausal fatigue and irritability are behind many of them.

Doctors from Well Men centers from all around Australia emphasize the important part that lack of testosterone can play in the rising level of depression and suicide that has been observed recently in Australia, and believe that hormone levels should be measured in men with the characteristic symptoms.

However, even on this visit in 1998, although there were encouraging signs of many more doctors being interested in the diagnosing and treating andropause, there were storm clouds on the horizon in the form of increasing opposition to the treatment from both academic and political sources.

The backlash

In August 1999 the backlash to the previous modest advances in the availability of testosterone treatment for andropause in Australia really set in. Until then the treatment had been available to men on subsidy under the Pharmaceutical Benefits Scheme (PBS) where, in the doctor's opinion, the man was 'hypogonadal.' This diagnosis was reached by the doctor from consideration of the man's presenting symptoms and supported by reference to pathology results from blood tests.

At that time most laboratories would provide guidance to doctors defining the reference of serum (total) testosterone of 11–35 nmols as being 'within normal range.' So if a man was at the lower end of the range and certainly if he was off the bottom end of the scale, and he had the characteristic symptoms of andropause, then doctors could obtain an authority prescription for testosterone replacement medication on subsidy under the PBS.

In fact, because most Australian GP's have received little or no formal training in the diagnosis or management of andropause, relatively few doctors were even considering hormones as a possible causative factor in erection problems, fatigue and depresson, so few diagnostic investigations were taking place, and only a small but rising number of prescriptions for testosterone were being requested.

Suddenly on August 1, 1999, the Australian government, with the encouragement and support of a small pressure group of academic endocrinologists, changed the ground rules in a way which denied the vast majority of men in that country any chance of getting testosterone treatment. The new rules were intended to increase restriction on access to hormone supplementation, for men only, and removed any role for the man's treating doctor in diagnosing his condition, as well as eliminating consideration of a man's symptoms entirely.

Instead, the government introduced rigid biochemical criteria whereby two morning blood samples, taken on different mornings, must show total testosterone levels of 8 nmols/l (230ng/dl) or less for a man to qualify for subsidy on medication under the PBS.

This restriction is totally against the international swing towards diagnosing testosterone deficiency on the basis of the characteristic symptoms it causes, and in cases of doubt, giving a therapeutic trial of the hormone, in preference to arbitrary, limited, and often inaccurate laboratory data. Because of all the reasons given earlier in this book for preferring measurements of free, active testosterone to the total hormone levels, and the fact that the High-T male only feels and functions well on high levels of the hormone, this piece of legislation can be considered as medically entirely inappropriate and regressive.

When forewarned of this change in the PBS regulations in June 1999, Linda and Dr Zentner, the prime movers in STAG, which by then had changed its name to 'Time for Men,' started in vain to protest to the Federal Government Medical Services. They argued, and continue to argue in an ongoing series of high profile court cases, that this legislation breaches the Sexual Discrimination Act, The International Covenant on Civil and Political Rights, and the Administrative Decisions (Judicial Review Act) 1977.

This is heavy legal stuff, and expensive to prove in court against entrenched governmental and medical opposition. Undaunted, the Time for Men team, including Linda, her business partner and national sports coach, Mike Ellis, and a representative group of men diagnosed as having had testosterone deficiency, together with their treating doctors led by Dr Zentner, are prepared to 'go to the wire' in trying to get this legislation reversed. Real-life David and Goliath stuff, but with very serious consequences for a million or more Australian men.

In effect, these men are being denied access to subsidized treatment for what many doctors, obviously myself included, strongly believe to be a true hormonal disorder, damaging every aspect of their physical, mental and social well-being. By contrast, an Aussie woman only has to go halfway down the list of symptoms before she is offered a trial of subsidized HRT and then if she gets symptoms, relief can continue on subsidized treatment. Not so the men – even if they have recovered completely on treatment given before the prescribing rules were changed, no carryover of benefit is allowed, and many of them have crashed horribly. The Australian government spent $30AU million on women's HRT last year and a miserly $3AU million on male HRT, which covered all causes of low testosterone in men, including the congenital ones. If, on the basis of the evidence presented in this book, there is an equivalent need, then this is an unjustified economy. Certainly it's a saving, but at what a huge cost to the men and their families suffering the consequences.

Details of this ongoing heroic struggle can be found on the web sites and national and international organizations listed in the 'Resources' section at the end of this book. Rather than being just a passive spectator in this fight against an obvious injustice, there is an opportunity for you to join in and help this beleaguered band of heroes in the testosterone revolution by providing financial, political, legal or medical support.

Let's now look at the timing of this testosterone revolution, and why there was this dramatic about face by the generals of orthodox opinion between two World Congresses, the First and Second meetings of the International Society for the Study of the Aging Male.

Chapter eleven

The testosterone revolution

After a lapse of more than half a century, the tide of medical and public opinion is turning rapidly towards acceptance of andropause as a true hormonal deficiency which can and should be treated with testosterone. Let's examine how this change has come about, and the ways in which the year 2000 became what I call 'the year of the testosterone revolution.'[1]

These revolutionary ideas are sweeping the world and are not just a localized event in any one country, although there are some notable exceptions, such as Australia, as already described. This can be seen in the major shift in medical opinion which happened in the period between two conferences sponsored by the World Health Organization, and held in Geneva in 1998 and 2000.

First World Congress on the Aging Male – 1998

The First World Congress on the Aging Male in February 1998, was organized by a very dynamic and farsighted Israeli physician and gynecologist, Professor Bruno Lunenfeld, president of the International Society for the Study of the Aging male and Editor in Chief of the 'Aging Male' journal which he started that year. This journal has rapidly become the key reference source and is compulsive reading for all those interested in the world view of men's health, and the important part testosterone can play in treatment and preventive medicine.

As he said in a call to arms at that first conference:

The conventional approach of the medical, behavioral and social sciences to the problem of male aging has been for a long time, the subject of oversight, absence of focusing, disconnection and, most of all, lack of interdisciplinary collaboration.

To correct these failings he assembled for the first time at any international conference a mixture of andrologists, gynecologists, urologists, gerontologists and general physicians from 35 countries who gave over 120 papers on a wealth of subjects. As could be seen from the conference proceedings, many of the speakers were either ultra-cautious or even hostile to the concept of andropause. They also expressed fear of the possible side effects of testosterone treatment, especially in relation to possible problems with the prostate and were unsure about the indications for its use. Everyone seemed to be hedging their bets, and not wanting to be seen to stick their necks out.

When I gave a paper on 'HRT for the aging male – A clinical study in 1,100 men' and dared to suggest

This form of HRT with testosterone may come to be considered as important a part of preventive medicine in the second half of life for men as estrogen is for women[2]

there was a little polite applause, and then hard hitting criticism from two of the academic scientists present, one from Australia and one from America. The Australian critic said that as my study was not a double blind, placebo cross-over trial, the paper should never have been given. I protested in vain that although I realized the short-comings of the paper, I thought that my detailed observations on the safety and effectiveness of three different types of testosterone treatment in 1,000 men over a period of eight years might be of interest to the more open-minded delegates I expected at that sort of innovative conference.

The American academician then leapt to his feet and joined in the attack on the paper's scientific shortcomings, making it clear that he didn't believe there was such a thing as the 'male menopause.' He suggested that I was creating an expensive and dangerous delusion in treating this mythical condition with testosterone.

On the last day of the conference he went on with this line of attack in his keynote lecture, and in an emotional rather than scientific critique, showed the cover of my original 'Male Menopause' book published two years earlier, among several he honored on a naming and trashing basis. Fortunately in doing so he made it clear he probably had not actually read any of them thoroughly, if at all, and had judged them largely on their covers. He also appeared to entirely confuse the terms 'male menopause' and 'male mid-life crisis,' and so was able to have a field day at the expense of those who he clearly regarded as charlatans, the doctors who tried to help men with symptoms they thought might indicate testosterone deficiency.

Despite this disappointing end to the conference, the assembled delegates, again skillfully steered by Professor Lunenfeld toward the broader view, drafted a 'Centennial Prospective – Healthy Aging for Men.' This predicted the rapid rise in the number of men over the age of 65 in many parts of the world, to over 25 percent of the male population in some countries within the decade. It considered that this would raise major social, economic and ethical issues worldwide, and might strain the health, socio-economic and even political infrastructures of many countries to the limit.

Therefore, it was suggested that the promotion of healthy aging and the prevention, or drastic reduction, of morbidity and disability of the elderly must assume a central role in the formation of the health and social policies of many, if not all, countries in the next century. The report included in its recommendations that obtaining information on men regarding interventions, such as hormone replacement therapy, which may favorably influence many of the diseases associated with male aging, as had been shown in women, was an 'urgent need.'

Second World Congress on the Aging Male – 2000

The climate of opinion at the second world congress was very different, especially towards andropause, and my previously expressed heretical views. Reflecting this change was the presence of several additional sponsors of the congress, including not only five major pharmaceutical companies who were waking up to the huge potential market in male HRT, but also academic bodies, including The European Association of Urology, The World Association of Sexology, and the European Menopause Society, which had just changed its name to the European Menopause and Andropause Society.

Again, the emphasis was on the WHO 'Aging and Health Program,' with the stated goal of promoting 'health and well-being throughout the lifespan, thus insuring the attainment of the best possible quality of life for as long as possible, for the largest possible number of older people.' As an important part of this drive, there were many more papers directly supporting testosterone treatment, and reporting good results and a high level of safety with it.

The best overall view of this was probably given by the interactive voting session organized and sponsored by Ferring AG Pharmaceutical company. The jury, 400 leading experts in the field, mainly urologists, endocrinologists, gynecologists and research scientists from all over the world, invited to a symposium called 'Testosterone Deficiency as a Real Clinical Issue in the Aging Male Population,' came out overwhelmingly in favor of testosterone treatment being important and beneficial. The questions put to them, and the answers they gave are reported in detail because they show a huge change in medical views on the theory and practice of the diagnosis and treatment of andropause.

Given electronic vote recorders for instant analysis of their views, they were asked the following ten key questions:

What do you consider a subnormal testosterone level?

Given a choice of 4, 8 and 12 nmol/l, the vote split evenly between the three levels, with a slight preference for the highest. Any clinician who could recognize the units would never have chosen the lowest level, as that would be grossly subnormal, the only real area of debate being between the upper two. This confusion may have resulted from the schism between units of measurement used in different countries. Many of the large contingent of U.S. and Canadian delegates were unable to equate 12 nmol/l total testosterone, the more favored lower limit of 'normal' in Europe, with the level of 350 ng/dl used by doctors trained in North America.

What are the most important symptoms of testosterone deficiency in men over 50?

The symptoms rated by the delegates as being most common were, in decreasing order of importance, loss of libido, erectile dysfunction, depression, reduced cognitive function, osteoporosis and reduced muscle strength. It is interesting that this vote by an authoritative body of expert opinion from all round the world should recognize exactly the same frequency of characteristic symptoms of androgen deficiency as I found in a detailed comparison of these in studies ranging from Dr August Werner in 1946,[3] to those reported in a study of web patients using the Andropause Check List given in chapter two.[4] This consistency of the clinical features of andropause, as observed by doctors all over the world for more than fifty years, further validates the importance of low testosterone levels in causing the condition,[5] and the validity of this questionnaire in its diagnosis.

What is the most appropriate way of diagnosing testosterone deficiency?

A large majority of the experts felt that characteristic symptoms must be present as well as subnormal testosterone levels, rather than reduced levels alone, with raised pituitary gonadotrophins being the least essential. This is a most important point as the purpose of testosterone treatment is to relieve symptoms, and the reason why men with andropausal symptoms, even with borderline laboratory findings, should be offered a therapeutic trial with adequate doses of the hormone for at least three months.

Do you prescribe testosterone replacement to men over 50?

Over 80 percent were currently prescribing testosterone to their male patients, and that presumably didn't include the gynecologists, who are also increasingly using small doses of testosterone in addition to HRT with estrogens in their female menopausal patients, to boost libido and well-being.

Which testosterone therapy do you prescribe to men over 50?

Pills were used by around 60 percent, intra-muscular injections by over 50 percent, transdermal body or scrotal patches by only about 10 percent each, and pellet implants by less than five percent. This suggests that men find patches inconvenient and irritating, and injections are the main form of testosterone treatment in the USA, where unlike in Canada, Europe, and most of the rest of the world, safe oral forms of testosterone are not yet available, although hopefully this will soon change.

Which testosterone therapy do these patients prefer?

Pills followed by injections were by far the most favored forms of treatment. This coincides with my clinical experience that scrotal and body patches are inconvenient to use, can easily fall off, and tend to irritate the skin. They also seem to deliver lower testosterone dosage, and suppress the body's own production more than oral treatments, although not as much as injections or implants. Also, compared to sixty years of safe and convenient use of pellet implants of testosterone, these newer methods have relatively little 'track-record' in terms of safety and efficiency in relieving andropausal symptoms long-term. All these reasons may be why Ferring AG stopped actively marketing their patches after this symposium, although we must be grateful to them for the interesting information gained from the ballot they sponsored at this conference.

What are the most important considerations when choosing which type of testosterone treatment to prescribe?

Effective symptom relief was most highly rated at nearly 35 percent, with ease of use, convenience, and examination for pre-existing disease at around 25 percent each, and cost, lifestyle and availability at less than 10 percent each. While recognizing the overriding importance of the first of these, because in most state medical systems availability is limited by cost, most patients describe the high price of most testosterone preparations as being the limiting factor in taking up this form of treatment.

Where do you stand on concern about potential risk of prostatic disease?

The responses to this question were most reassuring to doctors and patients alike. Over 75 percent of delegates said they would start treatment, but carefully monitor the PSA, 15 percent thought the potential benefits outweighed the potential risks, six percent would await the outcome of stringent risk versus benefit analyses and only two percent would not consider prescribing it because of the concerns about prostatic disease. These views coincided with good news from other speakers at the conference about prostate safety. These included papers by Professor Herman Behre from Germany and Stefan Arver from Sweden reporting detailed clinical studies on a variety of testosterone treatments, without adverse effects on the prostate.[6-7]

Where do you stand on concern about potential risk of cardiovascular disease?

This was again reassuring, especially for doctors who had been told from medical school onward that testosterone was bad for the heart. Nearly 70 percent were confident that the potential benefits outweighed the risks, less than 30 percent wanted to await the outcome of more stringent risk/benefit analysis, and only three percent would not consider prescribing it because of concerns about cardiovascular disease. The safety of testosterone treatment in relation to the circulation was reinforced by two other speakers from London at the conference; Dr Peter Collins,[8] who reported that testosterone dilates the coronary arteries, and Dr David Crook,[9] who reviewed the data on its relationship with heart attack risk factors, and found evidence of benefit rather than harm.

Do you consider there is sufficient evidence to initiate testosterone therapy for decreased bone mineral density in aging men?

Nearly 75 percent did think there was sufficient evidence to initiate treatment for osteoporotic aging males. This view was supported at the conference by another speaker, Dr Jean Kaufman from Ghent,

Belgium, who reported on studies suggesting a beneficial effect of reducing osteoporosis in men with low testosterone by giving HRT.[10]

These views represented a dramatic shift of opinion in favor of testosterone treatment even over the two years since the First World Congress on the Aging Male was held in Geneva. At the first conference, opinions had been much more evenly divided between those in favor and those wishing for a lot more evidence before they would consider treating their patients with testosterone.

The most important point about the second Congress is that the majority of experts seemed to think that evidence had been produced to their satisfaction, and they now felt confident about beginning treatment. The jury of international experts had considered the extensive evidence, and returned a verdict very much in favor of testosterone treatment.

The web-based revolution

Another interesting and increasingly important way of monitoring the progress of the testosterone revolution is via the World Wide Web, and this has become a powerful agent in its spread. It not only gives you instant access to news and views on testosterone treatment on a global basis, but can give you the latest medical publications in a very convenient and easily retrievable form. Some of the most useful of these web sites are listed in the resources section at the end of the book.

Web-medicine is increasingly seen as part of the move toward a world-wide solution to testosterone insufficiency in men in middle and later life. To make best use of scarce medical manpower and time, it is essential that the latest technology make all the relevant information about a patient easily accessible to physicians, in a secure electronic format, from which diagnostic and treatment decisions can economically be reached.

These principles have been applied to making patient data easily accessible to specialists working both in a clinic setting and via the Internet. Two web sites were created in the year 2000 to help with this problem, and have been operating successfully since.

The first, the www.androscreen.com screen provides a confidential and safe diagnostic service for patients anywhere in the world. It has been especially designed to help men with symptoms of andropause to get medical advice from the convenience and anonymity of their home computer terminal. Combined with a full laboratory profile, which can be obtained from over 1,000 Quest Diagnostic facilities in the USA alone, as well as throughout Europe, it can provide a detailed diagnostic report which the client can take to their local physician for advice and treatment.

The second site www.andropause.org.uk was set up by The Andropause Society (TAS). This is a newly established international charity with the aims of promoting the exchange of research information and ideas about Androgen Deficiency in the Adult Male (ADAM) between health professionals working in this field, and encouraging education and training about andropause and its treatment. It is hoped that doctors will join this new organization to extend the global network of over 1,000 physicians already recruited to make male HRT more easily available wherever the client lives.

Future of the testosterone revolution

The goal of a revolution is to bring about sustained change in a situation where natural evolution appears to be blocked, going too slowly for the common good, or even going in the wrong direction. Let's see what principles can be applied to insure a lasting future for the testosterone revolution.

Like most revolutions, it starts with the spark of creative fire from the leaders themselves who see the need for change. Even with the financial fuel in place, to fan the flames, to keep them burning, and have a lasting effect, there has to be a sustained effort on behalf of the leaders to keep its ideals spreading. Once the desired change has been brought about, it should have its own momentum so that it evolves and becomes part of the fabric of society. It can be seen to go through the phases of awareness of the need to change, action to achieve it, acceptance, and application once it has come about to insure it continues.

These phases can be seen in the thirty year war of estrogen treatment of female menopause. First, there was guerrilla action by a few isolated physicians who saw the need in some of their patients for this form of treatment. I worked with some of these in the sixties, mainly gynecologists who saw the onset of menopausal symptoms in their patients following hysterectomy, and the dramatic relief which could be obtained by giving HRT. I also saw the flack they received from doctors opposed to the treatment, who thought that it was against nature, and that women should learn to grow old gracefully without chemical intervention, and that it was dangerous to do otherwise.

This is equivalent to the early work of Drs Werner, Reiter and Møller described earlier, which was also met with skepticism and fierce antagonism from their colleagues, particularly in the groves of academia. The generals at medical headquarters did not think they had much to learn from the troops in the front line. What they, the experts, didn't know by definition and consensus wasn't worth knowing.

However, some of these pioneers persisted, and interested some of their more open-minded colleagues in moving from case reports to small-scale trials. The results of these were encouraging, and many patients, some of them high profile figures such as movie stars and actresses, were seen to be benefitting both in looks and vitality. They became walking advertisements for the treatment, and attracted much media attention, and created awareness of the possibilities for women generally.

The medical backlash however, was also strengthened by both increasing theoretical concerns about causing breast cancer, and by practical concerns about causing uterine cancer. However, this very practical problem was soon overcome for non-hysterectomized women by developing cyclical treatment with progesterone, although this did bring back periods in the women taking it. The benefits they experienced however seemed to make it worthwhile for the majority, although further more detailed research was obviously needed on the risk versus benefit equation.

Male HRT until recently seemed stuck at this phase of its evolution, and although there were sporadic attempts throughout the seventies and eighties to gain greater acceptance for the treatment, the general medical opinion was still very much against it. Female HRT began to attract much attention from the drug companies, who recognized the huge potential market for female HRT, and started funding the expensive large-scale studies needed for its full evaluation. However they did not see any such potential for equivalent treatment in the male, and that view was reinforced by the combined opposition of endocrine and urological opinion.

Indeed, this was an important part of the problem, because while women had attention from both their general practitioners and gynecologists, men were less demanding in seeking help, and had no real pressure group representing their special needs. This was particularly so in relation to a medical condition which didn't officially exist, particularly one which had acquired the derogatory title of male menopause.

While women's health was a real issue, and screening for breast and cervical cancer a real vote-grabber, men's health was not, and consequently attracted virtually no funds or research interest. The best example of this is the lack, up to now, of any publicly funded screening program for prostate cancer in the UK, compared to the far more active approach in the USA and Canada. While ten years ago, menopause groups were being formed in the UK and Europe, and world-wide gynecologists were bringing HRT into the routine treatment of postmenopausal women, men were experiencing the same symptoms but went untreated.

However, awareness of andropause is dawning among the public and among physicians world-wide. Progress, however, is very patchy as we have seen, ranging from an apparently high degree in Canada to very little in Australia. The World-Wide Web seems to offer a great opportunity for spreading information about the condition and the good news about its treatment. Also, the numbers of articles in mainstream medical journals is increasing exponentially as the concept infiltrates into a previously resistant culture.

Action is being taken by national organizations such as the Canadian Andropause Society, and international ones such as the International Society for the Study of the Aging Male (ISSAM) and its affiliates, especially in Asia. That ISSAM is supported by the World Health Organization is a sign of the growing realization by governments that promotion of well-being in a rapidly aging male population is not only socially and medical desirable, but economically essential.

To accelerate this change, new testosterone medications, and the research to back them, are needed to make treatment more effective, even safer, and above all cheaper to buy and apply. Above all, however, there is a need for training, especially of primary care physicians, in the basic skills of diagnosing andropause, and treating it with the testosterone preparations that are already available. This is neither brain surgery nor rocket science, and if it is to be applied to the mass of men who could benefit from it, cannot be limited to special clinics, although there will always be a place for these as with female HRT.

Again, the Canadian Andropause Society leads the way in its development of a training program for family physicians across Canada and for affiliated societies world-wide. The Andropause Society, based in the UK is hoping to take part in this initiative, and, if possible, help to make it available to a growing network of doctors in every country via the web, with a mixture of printed publicationss, web-casts and video-conferences. In these ways, the key information needed to apply male HRT effectively and safely could soon be coming to a physician's computer screen near you.

After all, it is the widespread application of this knowledge which is the ultimate goal of the testosterone revolution. What would be the use of doctors world-wide throwing their hands in the air and saying they agree that many men can suffer andropausal symptoms, which can and should be treated, and then doing nothing about it.

Lasting change needs continuous progress on all these fronts of awareness, action, acceptance and application, which is what this book is all about.

Long live the testosterone revolution for the benefit of all mankind.

References

Introduction: The male menopause mystery

1 Sheehy, G., *New Passages*. London: HarperCollins, 1996
2 Sheehy, G., 'Is there a male menopause?' *Vanity Fair* 1993; 164
3 Goldman, B., Klatz, R., *Death in the Locker Room: Drugs and Sports*. Chicago, Illinois: Elite Sports Medicine Publications Inc., 1992
4 Korkia, P., Stimson, G. V., *Anabolic Steroid Use in Great Britain: An exploratory investigation*. London: HMSO, 1993
5 Lunenfeld, B., 'An aging world – challenges ahead' *Aging Male* 2000; 4: 3–6
6 Hooper, R., *Medical Dictionary*. London: Murray and Highley, 1798
7 Werner, A. A., 'The Male Climacteric.' *J. Am. Med. Ass.* 1939; 112: 1441–3
8 Heller, C. G., Myers, G. B., 'The male climacteric: Its symptomatology, diagnosis and treatment' *JAMA* 1944; 126: 472
9 Editorial, ibid.
10 de Kruif, P., *The Male Hormone: A new gleam of hope for prolonging man's prime of life*. New York: Harcourt, Brace and Company, 1945
11 Skolnick, A. A., 'Is "male menopause" real or just an excuse?' *JAMA* 1994

Chapter one: The testosterone story

1 Medvei, V. C., *A History of Endocrinology*. Lancaster, England: MTP Press Ltd, 1982
2 de Kruif, P., *The Male Hormone: A new gleam of hope for prolonging man's prime of life*. New York: Harcourt, Brace and Company, 1945
3 Hamalainen, E., Adlercreutz, H., Puska, P., Pietinen, P., 'Diet and serum sex hormones in healthy men' *J Steroid Biochem* 1984; 20 (1): 459–64
4 Irvine, W., 'John Hunter's Experiments: Evidence of an eye witness. Letter to Professor Thomas Hamilton, University of Glasgow, of 17 June 1771' *Lancet* 1928; 359–60

5 Berthold, A. A., 'Transplantation der Hoden' *Arch Anat Physiol Wiss Med* 1849; 42–6

6 Medvei, op. cit.

7 Editorial, 'The pentacle of rejuvenescence *BMJ* 1889; 1:1416

8 de Kruif, op. cit.

9 Wright, S., *Applied Physiology*. London: Oxford Medical Publications, 1926

10 Ibid.

11 David, K., Dingemanse, E., Freud, J., Laqueur, E., 'Über krystallinisches männliches Hormon aus Hoden (Testosteron), wirksamer als aus Harn oder aus Cholesterin bereitetes Androsteron' *Hoppe-Seylers Z Physiol Chem* 1935; 233: 282

12 Butenandt, F. J., 'Über die chemische Untersuchung der Sexual-hormone' *Z Angew Chem* 1931; 44: 905–8

13 Butenandt, F. J., Hanish, G., 'Über Tesosteron. Umwanlung des Dehydro-androsterons in Androstendiol und Testosteron: ein Weg zur Darstellung des Testosterons aus Cholesterin' *Hoppe-Seylers Z Physiol Chem* 1935; 237: 89–98

14 Ruzicka, L., Wettstein, A., 'Synthetische Darstellung der Testishhormons, Testosteron (Androsten 3 on 17-ol)' *Helv Chim Acta* 1935; 18: 1264–75

15 Thomas, H. B., Hill, R. T., 'Testosterone propionate and the male climacteric' *Endocrinology* 1940; 26: 953

16 Deansley, R., Parkes, A. S., 'Further experiments on the administration of hormones by the subcutaneous implantation of tablet' *Lancet* 1938; 2: 606–8

17 Handelsman, D., 'Pharmacology of testosterone pellet implants' in Nieschlag, E., Behre, H. M., eds, *Testosterone: Action, deficiency, substitution*. Heidelberg: Springer Verlag, 1990; 136–54

18 Ruzicka, L., Goldburg, M. W., Rosenburg, H. R., 'Herstellung des 17-methyl-testosterons und anderer Androsten- und Androstanderivative zusammen' *Z P* 1935

19 Nieschlag, E., Behre, H. M., 'Pharmacology and clinical uses of testosterone' in Nieschlag, op. cit., 92–114

20 Heller, C. G., Myers, G. B., 'The male climacteric: Its symptomatology, diagnosis and treatment' *JAMA* 1944; 126: 472–77

21 Reiter, T., 'Treatment of male climacteric by combined implantation' *Practitioner* 1953; 170: 181

22 Reiter, T., 'Testosterone implantation: A clinical study of 240 implantations in ageing males' *Journal of the American Geriatrics Society* 1963; 11: 540–50

23 Reiter, T., 'Testosterone therapy' *British Journal of Geriatric Practice* 1967; 4 (2): 137–40

24 Reiter, T., *Reiter's Treatment of Testosterone Deficiency*. London: Organon Laboratories Ltd, 1965

25 Carruthers, M., Murray, A., *F/40: Fitness on Forty Minutes a Week*. London: Futura, 1976

26 Christiansen, J., *The Tvedegaard-Møller Trial: A fight against injustice*. Copenhagen: Rosenhilde and Begger, 1960

27 Møller, J., Einfeldt, H., *Testosterone Treatment of Cardiovascular Diseases*. Berlin, Springer Verlag, 1984

28 Møller, J., *Cholesterol: Interactions with testosterone and cortisol in cardiovascular disease*. Berlin: Springer Verlag, 1987

29 Møller, J., *Toxic oral antibiotics in relation to cardiovascular disease*. Munich: ECOMED, 1988

Chapter two: The male menopause or andropause

1 Carruthers, M., 'Diagnosis and treatment of the andropause' 2000. Proceedings of The Andropause Society, 1st annual conference, 12-6-2000

2 Bancroft, J., *Human Sexuality and its Problems*. Edinburgh: Churchill Livingstone, 1989

3 Bremner, C., 'Hormone count at root of lawyers' machismo' *Times Tribune*, 9 November 1990

4 Gladue, B. A., 'Aggressive behavioral characteristics, hormones, and sexual orientation in men and women' *Aggressive Behaviour* 1991; 17: 314–26

5 Baucom, D. H., 'Relation between testosterone concentration, sex role identity, and personality among females' *Journal of Personality and Social Psychology* 1985; 48: 1218–26

6 Greer, G., *The Change*. London: Penguin Books, 1992

7 Vermeulen, A., 'Androgens in the ageing male' *Journal of Clinical Endocrinology and Metabolism* 1991; 73: 221–4

8 Lichtenstein, M. J., Yarnell, J. M., Elwood, P. C., *et al.*, 'Sex hormones, insulin, lipids, and prevalent ischemic heart disease' *American Journal of Epidemiology* 1987; 126 (4): 647–57

9 Barrett-Conner, E., Khaw, K., 'Endogenous sex hormones and cardiovascular disease in men: A prospective population-based study' *Circulation* 1988; 78: 539–44

10 Møller, J., Einfeldt, H., *Testosterone Treatment of Cardiovascular Diseases*. Berlin, Springer Verlag, 1984

11 Feldman, J. M., Postlethwaite, R. W., Glenn, J. F., 'Hot flashes and sweats in men with testicular insufficiency' *Arch Intern Med* 1976; 136: 606–8

12 Francis, R. M., Peacock, M., Aaron, J. E., *et al.*, 'Osteoporosis in hypogonadal men: Role of decreased plasma 1,25-dihydroxyvitamin D, calcium malabsorption, and low bone formation' *Bone* 1986; 7: 261–8

13 Kelly, P. J., *et al.*, 'Dietary calcium, sex hormones, and bone mineral density in men' *BMJ* 1990; 300: 1361–4

14 Phillips, S. K., *et al.*, 'Muscle weakness in women occurs at an earlier age than in men, but strength is preserved by hormone replacement therapy' *Clinical Science* 1993; 84: 95–8

Chapter three: Not the mid-life crisis

1 Brim, O. G., 'Theories of the male mid-life crisis' *Counselling Psychologist* 1976; 6: 2–9
2 Amis, M., *The Information*. London: HarperCollins, 1995
3 Dimbleby, J., *The Prince of Wales: A biography*. London: Little, Brown & Co., 1994
4 Lax, E., *Woody Allen: A biography*. London: Jonathan Cape, 1991
5 Barrymore, M., *Back in Business*. London: Hutchinson, 1995
6 Lewis, R., *The Life and Death of Peter Sellers*. London: Century, 1994
7 Davis, J. H., *The Kennedys: Dynasty and disaster 1848–1983*. New York: McGraw-Hill, 1984
8 Markson, E. W., Gognalons, N. M., 'Midlife: Crisis or nodal point?' in Hess, B., Markson, E. W., eds, *Growing Old in America*. New Brunswick, NJ: Transaction, 1991
9 Jaques, E., 'Death and the mid-life crisis' *Int J Psycho-analysis* 1965; 46: 502–14
10 Carruthers, M., *The Western Way of Death: Stress, tension and heart disease*. London and New York: Davis-Poynter and Pantheon Books, 1974

Chapter four: How it happens

1 Moir, A., Jessel, D., *Brain Sex*. London: Michael Joseph, 1989
2 Gray, A., Jackson, D. N., McKinlay, J. B., 'The relation between dominance, anger and hormones in normally aging men: Results from the Massachusetts male aging study' *Psychosomatic Medicine* 1991; 53: 374–85
3 Dabbs, J., De la Rue, D., Williams, P. M., 'Testosterone and occupational choice: Actors, ministers and other men' *Journal of Personality and Social Psychology* 1990; 59: 1261–5
4 Rommerts, F. F. G., 'Testosterone: An overview of biosynthesis, transport, metabolism and action' in Nieschlag, E., Behre, H. M., eds, *Testosterone: Action, deficiency, substitution*. Heidelberg: Springer Verlag, 1990; 1–22
5 Hamalainen, E., Adlercreutz, H., Puska, P., Pietinen, P., 'Diet and serum sex hormones in healthy men' *J Steroid Biochem* 1984; 20 (1): 459–64
6 Carruthers, M., *The Western Way of Death: Stress, tension and heart disease*. London and New York: Davis-Poynter and Pantheon Books, 1974
7 Rudman, D., Feller, A. G., Nagraj, H. S., *et al.*, 'Effects of human growth hormone in men over 60 years old' *New England Journal of Medicine* 1990; 323 (1): 1–6

8 Vermeulen, A., 'Androgens and male senescence' in Nieschlag, E., Behre, H. M., eds, *Testosterone: Action, deficiency, substitution.* Heidelberg: Springer Verlag, 1990; 261–76

9 Schmidt, H., Starcevic, Z., 'Urinary testosterone excretion in men at different ages and the causation of testicular insufficiency' *Klin Wschr* 1967; 45: 377–82

10 Neaves, W. B., Johnson, L., Porter, I. C., Parker, C. R., Petty, C. S., 'Leydig cell numbers, daily sperm production and serum gonadotrophin levels in aging men' *J Clin Endocrinol Metab* 1984; 59: 756–63

11 Sparrow, D., Boss, R., Rowe, J. N., 'The influence of age, alcohol consumption and body build on gonadal function in men' *J Clin Endocrinol Metab* 1980; 51: 508–12

12 Plymate, S. R., Tenover, J. S., Bremner, W. J., 'Circadian variations in testosterone, sex hormone binding globulin testosterone in healthy young and elderly men' *J Androl* 1989; 10: 366–71

13 Sharpe, R. M., Skakkebaek, N. E., 'Are oestrogens involved in falling sperm counts and disorders of the male reproductive tract?' *Lancet* 1993; 341: 1392–5

14 Sharpe, R. M., 'Another DDT connection' *Nature* 1995; 374: 538–9

15 Toppari, J., et al., 'Male reproductive health and environmental chemicals with estrogenic effects' 1995; Miljoprojekt 290: 1–166

16 Carruthers, M., 'The case of the caponized farmers' *Back to Nature* British Andrology Society, 1995

17 Dodds, E. C., Golberg, L., Lawson, W., Robinson, R., 'Oestrogenic activity of certain synthetic compounds' *Nature* 1938; 141: 247–8

18 Dodds, E. C., Golberg, L., Lawson, W., Robinson, R., 'Oestrogenic activity of alkylated stilboestols' *Nature* 1938; 142: 34

19 Kelce, W. R., Stone, C. R., Laws, S. C., Gray, E. L., Kemppainen, J. A., Wilson, E. M., 'Persistent DDT metabolite *p.p*'-DDE is a potent androgen receptor antagonist' *Nature* 1995; 375: 581–5

20 Steinberger, E., 'The etiology and pathophysiology of testicular dysfunction in man' *Fertil Steril* 1978; 29: 481–91

21 Wolnisty, C., 'Orchitis as a complication of infectious mononucleosis' *New England Journal of Medicine* 1962; 266: 88

22 Hubert, W., 'Psychotropic effects of testosterone' in Nieschlag, E., Behre, H. M., eds, *Testosterone: Action, deficiency, substitution.* Heidelberg: Springer Verlag, 1990; 51–71

23 Arguelles, A. E., Carruthers, M. E., Mosovich, A., 'Man in transit: Biochemical and physiological changes during intercontinental flights' *Lancet* 1976; 1: 977–81

24 Poggi, U. L., Arguelles, A. E., Rosner, J., et al., 'Plasma testosterone and serum lipids in male survivors of myocardial infarction' *Journal of Steroid Biochemistry* 1976; 7: 229–31

25 Kreuz, L. E., Rose, R. M., Jennings, J. R., 'Suppression of plasma testosterone levels and psychological stress' *Arch Gen Psychiat* 1972; 26: 479–82

26 Mazur, A., Lamb, T. A., 'Testosterone, status and mood in human males' *Horm Behav* 1980; 14: 236–46

27 Fox, C. A., Ismail, A. A., Love, D. N., Kirkham, K. E., Loraine, J. A., 'Studies on the relationship between plasma testosterone levels and human sexual activity' *J Endocrinol* 1996; 52: 51–8

28 Mathur, R. S., Neff, M. R., Landgreve, S. C., 'Time-related changes in the plasma concentrations of prolactin, gonadotrophins, sex hormone binding globulin, and certain steroid hormones in female runners after a long distance race' *Fertil Steril* 1986; 6: 1067–70

29 Van Thiel, D., Lester, R., 'The effect of chronic alcohol abuse on sexual function' *Clinics in Endocrinology and Metabolism* 1979; 8: 499–510

30 Sparrow, *et al.*, op. cit.

31 Cornaro, L., *Sure Methods of Attaining a Long and Healthfull Life*. 1530

32 Ando, S., *et al.*, 'The influence of age on Leydig cell function in patients with varicocele' *Int J Androl* 1996; 7: 104–18

33 Parazzini, F., *et al.*, 'Tight underpants and trousers and risk and dyspermia' *Int J Androl* 1995; 18: 137–40

Chapter five: Vasectomy: the unkindest cut of all

1 Goldstein, M., Feldberg, M., *The Vasectomy Book: A complete guide to decision making*. Wellingborough, Northamptonshire: Turnstone Press, 1985

2 Ibid.

3 Wolfers, D., Wolfers, H., *Vasectomy and Vasectomania*. London: Mayflower Books Ltd, 1974

4 Hodgekinson, N., 'It's Safer to Wait' *Daily Mail*, 4 April 1979

5 Nirapathpongporn, A., Huber, D. H., Krieger, J. N., 'No-scalpel vasectomy at the King's birthday vasectomy festival' *Lancet* 1990; 335: 894–5

6 McMahon, A. J., Buckley, J., Taylor, A., Lloyd, S. N., Deane, R. F., Kirk, D., 'Chronic testicular pain following vasectomy' *Br J Urol* 1992; 69: 188–91

7 Chen, T. F., Ball, R. Y., 'Epididymectomy for post-vasectomy pain: Historical review' *Br J Urol* 1991; 68: 407–13

8 Fowler, J. E. Jr., Mariano, M., 'Immunoglobulin in seminal fluid of fertile, infertile, vasectomy and vasectomy reversal patients' *J Urol* 1983; 129: 869–72

9 Isidori, A., Dondero, F., Lenzi, A., 'Immunobiology of male infertility' *Hum Reprod* 1988; 3: 75–7

10 Flickinger, C. J., Herr, J. C., Howards, S. S., *et al.*, 'Early testicular changes after vasectomy and vasovasostomy in Lewis rats' *Anat Rec* 1990; 227: 37–46

11 Flickinger, C. J., Howards, S. S., Carey, P. O., *et al.*, 'Testicular alterations are linked to the presence of elevated antisperm antibodies in Sprague-

Dawley rats after vasectomy and vasovasostomy' *J Urol* 1988; 140: 627–31

12 Rommerts, F. F. G., 'Testosterone: An overview of biosynthesis, transport, metabolism and action' in Nieschlag, E., Behre, H. M., eds, *Testosterone: Action, deficiency, substitution*. Heidelberg: Springer Verlag, 1990; 1–22

13 Petty, R., 'Serum testosterone, vasectomy and erectile dysfunction: A study' *RCGP Members Reference Handbook*, 1995; 281–3

14 Fawcett, D. W., Howards, S. S., Kisker, T., Alexander, N., Clarksen, T. B., *Vasectomy: Immunologic and pathophysiologic effects in animals and man*. New York: Academic Press, 1979

15 Glavind, K., Lauritsen, N. R., Klove-Mogensen, M., Carl, J., 'The effect of vasectomy on the production of plasma luteinizing hormone and follicle stimulating hormone in man' *Int Urol Nephrol* 1990; 22: 553–9

16 Peng, X. S., Li, F. D., Miao, Z. R., *et al.*, 'Plasma reproductive hormones in normal and vasectomized Chinese males' *Int J Androl* 1987; 10: 471–9

17 John, E., *et al.*, 'Vasectomy and prostate cancer: Results from a multi-ethnic case-control study' *Journal of the National Cancer Institute* 1995; 87 – N 9: 662–9

18 Strader, C. H., Weiss, N. S., Daling, J. R., 'Vasectomy and the incidence of testicular cancer' *Am J Epidemiol* 1988; 128: 56–63

19 Cale, A. R., Farouk, M., Prescott, R. J., Wallace, I. W., 'Does vasectomy accelerate testicular tumour? Importance of testicular examinations before and after vasectomy' *BMJ* 1990; 300: 370

20 Thornhill, J. A., Conroy, R. M., Kelly, D. G., Walsh, A., Fennelly, J. J., Fitzpatrick, J. M., 'An evaluation of predisposing factors for testis cancer in Ireland' *Eur Urol* 1988; 14: 429–33

21 Nienhuis, H., Goldacre, M., Seagroatt, V., Gill, L., Vessey, M., 'Incidence of disease after vasectomy: A record linkage retrospective cohort study' *BMJ* 192; 304: 743–6

22 Brown, L. M., Pottern, L. M., Hoover, R. N., 'Testicular cancer in young men: The search for causes of the epidemic increase in the United States' *J Epidemiol Community Health* 1987; 41: 349–54

23 Toppari, J., *et al.*, 'Male reproductive health and environmental chemicals with estrogenic effects' *Miljoprojekt* 1995; 290: 1–166

24 Rosenberg, L., Palmer, J. R., Zauber, A. G., Warshauer, M. E., Stolley, P. D., Shapiro, S., 'Vasectomy and the risk of prostate cancer' *American Journal of Epidemiology* 1990; 132: 1051–5

25 Peng, *et al.*, op. cit.

26 Møller, J., Einfeldt, H., *Testosterone Treatment of Cardiovascular Diseases*. Berlin: Springer Verlag, 1984

27 Howard, A. N., Patelski, J., Bowyer, D. E., Gresham, G. A., 'Atherosclerosis induced in hypercholesterolaemic by immunological injury; and the effects of intravenous polyunsaturated phosphatidyl choline' *Atherosclerosis* 1971; 14: 17–29

28 Alexander, N. J., Clarkson, T. B., 'Vasectomy increases the severity of diet-induced atherosclerosis in *Macaca fascicularis' Science* 1978; 201: 538–41

29 Anderson, K. M., Wilson, P. W., Garrison, R. J., Castelli, W. P., 'Longitudinal and secular trends in lipoprotein cholesterol measurements in a general population sample' The Framingham Offspring Study. *Atherosclerosis* 1987; 68: 59–66

30 Chi, I. C., Kong, S. K., Wilkens, L. R., *et al.*, 'Vasectomy and cardiovascular deaths in Korean men: A community-based case-control study' *Int J Epidemiol* 1990; 19; 1113–15

31 Petitti, D. B., Klein, R., Kipp, H., Friedman, G. D., 'Vasectomy and the incidence of hospitalized illness' *J Urol* 1983; 129: 760–2

32 Forti, G., Selli, C., 'Prospects for prostatic cancer incidence and treatment by the year 2000' *Int J Androl* 1996; 19: 1–10

33 Møller, op. cit.

34 Nienhuis, *et al.*, op. cit.

35 Forti, op. cit.

36 McDonald, S. W., 'Vasectomy and the human testis: We still know too little about the effects of vasectomy' Editorial, *BMJ* 1990; 301: 618–19

37 Cooper, A. P., *Observations on the Structure and Diseases of the Testis*. London: Longman, 1831; 51

Chapter six: Testosterone Replacement Therapy (TRT)

1 Forti, G., Selli, C., 'Prospects for prostatic cancer incidence and treatment by the year 2000' *Int J Androl* 1996; 19: 1–10

2 Rommerts, F. F. G., 'Testosterone: An overview of biosynthesis, transport, metabolism and action' in Nieschlag, E., Behre, H. M., eds, *Testosterone: Action, deficiency, substitution*. Heidelberg: Springer Verlag, 1990; 1–22

3 Joran, V. C., Murphy, C. S., 'Endocrine pharmacology of antiestrogens as antitumor agents' *Endocr Rev* 1990; 11: 578–610

4 Howell, A., DeFriend, D., Robertson, J., Blamey, R., Walton, P., 'Response to a specific antioestrogen (ICI 182780) in tamoxifen resistant breast cancer' *Lancet* 1995; 345: 29–30

5 Toppari, J., *et al.*, 'Male reproductive health and environmental chemicals with estrogenic effects' 1995; *Miljoprojekt* 290: 1–166

6 Nieschlag, E., Behre, H. M., 'Pharmacology and clinical uses of testosterone' in Nieschlag, E., Behre, H. M., eds, *Testosterone: Action, deficiency, substitution*. Heidelberg: Springer Verlag, 1990; 92–114

7 Heller, C. G., Myers, G. B., 'The male climacteric: Its symptomatology, diagnosis and treatment' *JAMA* 1944; 126: 472–77

8 Møller, J., Einfeldt, H., *Testosterone Treatment of Cardiovascular Diseases*. Berlin: Springer Verlag, 1984

9 Nieschlag, op. cit.

10 Handelsman, D. J., 'Pharmacology of testosterone pellet implants' in Nieschlag, E., Behre, H. M., eds, *Testosterone: Action, deficiency, substitution*. Heidelberg: Springer Verlag, 1990; 136–54

11 Jayle, M. F., 'In memoriam. Percutaneous absorption of steroids' in Mauvais-Jarvis, P., Vickers, C. F., Wepierre, J., eds, London: Academic Press, 1980; 273–83

12 Delanoe, D., Fougeyrollas, B., Meyer, L., Thonneau, P., 'Androgenisation of female partners of men on medroxyprogesterone acetate/percutaneous testosterone contraception' *Lancet* 1984; 4: 276–7

13 Place, V. A., Atkinson, L., Prather, D. A., Trunnell, N., Yates, F. E., 'Transdermal testosterone replacement through genital skin' in Nieschlag, E., Behre, H. M., eds, *Testosterone: Action, deficiency, substitution*. Heidelberg: Springer Verlag, 1990; 165–81

14 Bals-Pratsch, M., Knuth, U. A., Yoon, Y., Nieschlag, E., 'Transdermal testosterone substitution therapy for male hypogonadism' *Lancet* 1986; 2: 943–6

15 Mazer, N. S., *et al.*, 'Mimicking the circadian pattern of testosterone and metabolite levels with an enhanced transdermal delivery system' in Gurney, Junjinges, Peppas, eds, *Pulsatile Drug Delivery: Current applications and future trends*. Stuttgart: Niss. Verl. Ges. 1993; 73–97

16 Vermeulen, A., 'Androgens and male senescence' in Nieschlag, E., Behre, H. M., eds, *Testosterone: Action, deficiency, substitution*. Heidelberg: Springer Verlag, 1990; 261–76

17 Carruthers, M., *ADAM: Androgen Deficiency in the Adult Male: Causes, diagnosis and treatment*. New York: Parthenon Publishing, Inc., in press

18 Korkia, P. Stimson, G. V., *Anabolic Steroid Use in Great Britain: An exploratory investigation*. London: HMSO, 1993

19 Zhang, G.-Y., Li, G.-Z., Wu, F. W., Baker, H. G., Wang, X.-H., Soufir, J. C. *et al.*, 'Contraceptive efficacy of testosterone-induced azoospermia in normal men' *Lancet*, 1990; 336 (8721), pp. 955–959

20 Brendler, H., 'Endocrine regulation of prostatic growth' in Engle, E. T., Pincus, G., eds, *Hormones and the Aging Process*. New York: Academic Press Inc., 1956; 273

21 Schroder, F. H., 'Androgens and carcinoma of the prostate' in Nieschlag, E., Behre, H. M., eds, *Testosterone: Action, deficiency, substitution*. Heidelberg: Springer Verlag, 1990; 245–60

22 Sheehy, G., *The Silent Passage*. New York: Random House, 1993

23 Carruthers, M., 'More effective testosterone treatment: Combination with sildenafil and danazol' *The Aging Male* 2000; 14: 16

24 Kaufman, J. M., Vermeulen, A., 'Androgens in male senescence' in Nieschlag, E., Behre, H. M., eds, *Testosterone: Action, deficiency, substitution*. Berlin: Springer Verlag, 1990; 437–71

25 Longcope G., Feldman, H. A., McKinlay, J. B., Araujo, A. B., 'Diet and sex hormone-binding globulin' *J Clin Endocrinol Metab* 2000; 85: 293–6

Chapter seven: Sexual satisfaction

1 Bancroft, J., *Human Sexuality and its Problems*. Edinburgh: Churchill Livingstone, 1989
2 Ibid.
3 Toone, B. K., Wheeler, M., Nanjee, N., Fenwick, P., Grant, R., 'Sex hormones, sexual activity and plasma anticonvulsant levels in male epileptics' *Journal of Neurology, Neurosurgery and Psychiatry* 1983; 46: 824–6
4 Fenwick, P. B., Mercer, S., Grant, R., *et al.*, 'Nocturnal penile tumescence and serum testosterone levels' *Archives of Sexual Behaviour* 1986; 15: 13–22
5 Martin, L. M., 'Treatment of male sexual dysfunction with sex therapy' in Montague, D. K., ed., *Year Book 1988*. Chicago: Year Book Medical Publishers, 1988; 142–53
6 Masters, W. H., Johnson, V. E., *Human Sexual Inadequacy*. London: Churchill, 1970
7 Bancroft, op. cit.
8 Heller, C. G., Myers, G. B., 'The male climacteric: Its symptomatology, diagnosis and treatment' *JAMA* 1944; 126: 472–77
9 Huws, R., 'Antihypertensive medication and sexual problems' in Riley, A. J., Peet, M., Wilson, C., eds, *Sexual Pharmacology*. Oxford: Oxford University Press, 1993; 146–58
10 Barnes, T. R. E., Harvey, C. A., 'Psychiatric drugs and sexuality' in Riley, A. J., Peet, M., Wilson, C., eds, *Sexual Pharmacology*. Oxford: Oxford University Press, 1993; 176–96
11 Kaplan, H. S., *Disorders of Sexual Desire*. New York: Brunner Mazel Inc., 1979
12 Gomaa, A., *et al.*, 'Topical cream for erectile dysfunction: Randomised, double-blind placebo controlled trial of cream containing ammophylline, isosorbide dinitrate and co-dergocrine mesylate' *BMJ* 1996; 312: 1512–15

Chapter eight: Viagra and the magic gun

1 Harris, F., *My life and Loves* London: W. H. Allen, 1964
2 Feldman, H. A., Goldstein, I., Hatzichristou, D. G., Krane, R. J., McKinlay, J. B. 'Impotence and its medical and psychosocial correlates: Results of the Massachusetts Male Aging Study' *J Urol* 1994; 151: 54–61
3 Goldstein, I., Lue, T. F., Padma-Nathan, H., Rosen, R. C., Steers, W. D., Wicker, P. A. 'Oral sildenafil in the treatment of erectile dysfunction' Sildenafil Study Group. *N Engl J Med* 1998; 338: 1397–404
4 Palmer, R. M., Ferrige, A. G., Moncada, S. 'Nitric oxide release accounts for the biological activity of endothelium-derived relaxing factor' *Nature* 1987; 327: 524–6
5 Moncada, S., Palmer, R. M., Higgs, E. A., 'Nitric oxide: physiology, pathophysiology, and pharmacology' *Pharmacol Rev* 1991; 43: 109–42

6 Carruthers, M., 'Beyond Viagra: Combining testosterone and sildenafil for the treatment of erectile dysfunction.' 1998. Stamford CT. Conference Proceeding

7 Carruthers, M., 'More effective testosterone treatment: Combination with sildenafil and danazol' *Aging Male* 2000; 14: 16

8 Lugg, J., Ng, C., Rajfer, J., Gonzalez-Cadavid, N., 'Cavernosal nerve stimulation in the rat reverses castration-induced decrease in penile NOS activity' *Am J Physiol* 1996; 271: E354–E361

9 Gould, D. C., 'Combined testosterone and sildenafil treatment more effective than sildenafil alone' *Int J Impot Res* 1999; 11: 237–8

10 Gould, D. C., 'Efficacy of Viagra in hypogonadal men before and after testosterone replacement therapy' 2001. Proceedings of the 1st Conference Annual International Conference of The Andropause Society. 6-12-2000.

11 Carruthers, M., *The Western Way of Death: Stress, tension and heart disease.* London and New York: Davis-Poynter and Pantheon Books, 1974.

12 Shakir, S. A., Wilton, L. V., Boshier, A., Layton, D., Heeley, E., 'Cardiovascular events in users of sildenafil: results from first phase of prescription event monitoring in England' *BMJ* 2001; 322: 651–2

Chapter nine: Secrets of vitality and virility

1 Carruthers, M., 'Hormone replacement therapy for men' *RCGP Members Reference Book* 1993; 283–5

2 Carruthers, M., *The Western Way of Death: Stress, tension and heart disease.* London and New York: Davis-Poynter and Pantheon Books, 1974

3 Carruthers, M., 'Hypothesis: Aggression and atheroma' *Lancet* 1969; 2: 1170–1

4 Taggart, P., Parkinson, P., Carruthers, M. E., 'Cardiac responses to thermal, physical and emotional stress' *British Medical Journal* 1972; 3: 71–6

5 Carruthers, M. E., Taggart, P., 'Endogenous hyperlipidaemia induced by stress of racing driving' *Lancet* 1971; 1: 363–6

6 Friedman, M., Rosenman, R. H. *Type-A Behavior and your Heart.* New York, Alfred A. Knopf, 1972

7 Carter, J., *Nasty People: How to stop being hurt by them without becoming one of them.* Chicago: Contemporary Books, 1989

8 Byrne, E., *The Games People Play.* New York: Pantheon, 1974

9 Carruthers and Taggart, op. cit.

10 Ibid.

11 Poteliakhoff, A., Carruthers, M., *Real Health: The ill effects of stress and their prevention.* London: Davis-Poynter, 1981

12 Carruthers, M., Murray, A., *F/40: Fitness on Forty Minutes a Week.* London: Futura, 1976

13 Carruthers, M. E., 'Exercise programmes: The European experience' *British Journal of Sport and Medicine* 1979; 12: 235–40

14 Taggart, Parkinson and Carruthers, op. cit.

15 Carruthers, M., 'Voluntary control of the involuntary nervous system: Comparison of Autogenic Training and siddha meditation' in McGuigan, M. J., Sime, W. E., and Macdonald Wallace, J., eds, *Stress and Tension Control*. New York and London: Plenum Press, 1979; 267–75

16 Luthe, W., *Autogenic Therapy: Research and theory*. New York and London: Grune and Stratton, 1970

17 Carruthers, M. E., 'Autogenic Training' *J Psychosom Res* 1979; 23: 437–40

18 Hayes, P., *The Supreme Adventure*. London: Thorsons, 1995

19 Muktananda, S., *Meditate*. Albany: State University of New York Press, 1980

20 Diamond, J., *Male Menopause*. Naperville, Calif.: Sourcebooks Inc, 1997

21 Diamond, J., *The Warrior's Journey Home: Healing men, healing the planet*. Naperville, Calif.: Sourcebooks Inc, 1998

Chapter ten: Testosterone odyssey 2001

1 Werner, A. A., 'The male climacteric: Report of two hundred and seventy-three cases' *J Am Med Ass* 1946; 132: 188–94.

2 Heller, C. G., Myers, G. B., 'The male climacteric: Its symptomatology, diagnosis and treatment' *JAMA* 1944: 126; 472–7

3 Sevringhaus, E. L., *The Management of the Climacteric*. Illinois: Thomas, C.C., 1948

4 de Kruif, P., *The Male Hormone*. New York: Harcourt, Brace and Company, 1945

5 Swerdloff, R. S., Wang, C., 'Androgens, estrogens, and bone in men' *Ann Intern Med* 2000; 133: 1002–4

6 Hansen, M., 'Testosterone in the treatment of circulatory disease' 2000. The Andropause Society. Conference Proceeding 6-12-2000

7 Sheehy, G., *The Silent Passage*. London: HarperCollins, 1991

8 Sheehy, G., 'Is There a Male Menopause?' *Vanity Fair* (April), 164. 1993.

9 Sheehy, G., *New Passages: Mapping your life across time*. London: HarperCollins, 1996

10 McKinlay, J. B., Longcope, C., Gray, A., 'The questionable physiologic and epidemiologic basis for a male climacteric syndrome: Preliminary results from the Massachusetts Male Aging Study. *Maturitas* 1989; 11(2): 103–115

11 Longcope, C., Feldman, H. A., McKinlay, J. B., Araujo, A. B., 'Diet and sex hormone-binding globulin' *J Clin Endocrinol Metab* 2000; 85: 293–6

12 Araujo, A. B., Johannes, C. B., Feldman, H. A., Derby, C. A., McKinlay, J. B., 'Relation between psychosocial risk factors and incident erectile dysfunction: prospective results from the Massachusetts Male Aging Study' *Am J Epidemiol* 2000; 152: 533–41

13 Tenover, J. L. 'Testosterone replacement therapy in older adult men' *Int J Androl* 1999; 22: 300–6

14 Tenover, J. L., 'Male HRT in the new Millennium: An update' *Aging Male* 2000; 3: 4

15 Vermeulen, A., Stoica, T., Verdonck, L., 'The apparent free testosterone concentration, an index of androgenicity' *J Clin Endocrinol Metab* 1971; 33: 759–67

16 Kaufman, J. M., Vermeulen, A., 'Androgens in male senescence' in Nieschlag, E., Behre, H. M., eds, *Testosterone: Action, deficiency, substitution.* Berlin: Springer Verlag, 1998; 437–71

17 Leifke, E., Gorenoi, V., Wichers, C., Von Zur, M. A., Von Buren, E., Brabant, G., 'Age-related changes of serum sex hormones, insulin-like growth factor-1 and sex-hormone binding globulin levels in men: cross-sectional data from a healthy male cohort' *Clin Endocrinol (Oxf)* 2000; 53: 689–95

18 Gooren, L. J., 'A ten-year safety study of the oral androgen testosterone undecanoate' *J Androl* 1994; 15: 212–15

19 Gooren, L. G., 'Quality-of-life issues in the aging male' *Aging Male* 2000; 3: 185–9

20 Behre, H. M., 'Testosterone effects on the prostate' *Aging Male* 2000; 3: 5.

21 Gould, D. C., Petty, R., Jacobs, H. S., 'For and against: The male menopause – does it exist?' *BMJ* 2000; 320: 858–61

22 Gould, D. C., Petty, R., Jacobs, H. S., 'The male menopause – does it exist?' *Western Journal of Medicine* 2000; 173: 76–80

23 Tremblay, R. R., Morales, A. J., 'Canadian practice recommendations for screening, monitoring and treating men affected by andropause or partial androgen deficiency' *Aging Male* 1998; 1: 213–18

24 Tan, H. M., 'First Asian ISSAM Meeting: Managing aging populations – A global challenge' *Aging Male* 2001; 4

25 Carruthers, M., *Male menopause: Restoring vitality and virility* HarperCollins, London, 1996

Chapter eleven: The testosterone revolution

1 Carruthers, M., '2,000: The year of ADAM – The testosterone revolution' 2000. The Andropause Society WebCast. 6-12-2000.

2 Carruthers, M., 'HRT for the aging male: A clinical study in 1,000 men' *The Aging Male* 1998; 1: 34

3 Werner, A. A., 'The male climacteric: Report of two hundred and seventy three cases' *J Am Med Ass* 1946; 132: 188–94

4 Carruthers, M., 'ADAM: Androgen Deficiency in the Adult Male – causes, diagnosis and treatment' New York and Carnforth, Lancs.: The Parthenon Publishing Inc., in press

5   Tremblay, R. R., Morales, A. J., 'Canadian practice recommendations for screening, monitoring and treating men affected by andropause or partial androgen deficiency' *Aging Male* 1988; 1: 213–18

6   Behre, H. M., 'Testosterone effects on the prostate' *Aging Male* 2000; 3: 5

7   Meikle, A. W., Arver, S., Dobs, A. S., Adolfsson, J., Sanders, S. W., Middleton, R. G. *et al.*, 'Prostate size in hypogonadal men treated with a nonscrotal permeation-enhanced testosterone transdermal system' *Urology* 1997; 49: 191–6

8   Collins, P., 'Androgens and coronary artery disease: a case for protection?' *Aging Male 3* (WCAM Supplement). 11-2-2000. New York, London: Parthenon Publishing Group.

9   Godsland, I. F., Wynn, V., Crook, D., Miller, N. E., 'Sex, plasma lipoproteins, and atherosclerosis: prevailing assumptions and outstanding questions' *Am Heart J* 1987; 114: 1467–503

10 Kaufman, J. M., Vermeulen, A., 'Androgens in male senescence' in Nieschlag, E., Behre, H. M., eds, *Testosterone: Action, deficiency, substitution*. Berlin: Springer Verlag, 1998; 437–71

Resources

Web sites

The AndroScreen www.androscreen.com On-line diagnostic screening service and an internet web site set up to provide help for men who think they might be suffering from andropause. It is continually building up a network of doctors who are able to treat andropause. Physicians can apply to become part of the AndroScreen program by visiting the site.

The Andropause Society www.andropause.org.uk A UK-based charity, with the aims of promoting the exchange of research information and ideas about Androgen Deficiency in the Adult Male (ADAM) between health professionals working in this field, as well as to encourage education and training in andropause, its consequences and its treatment

The Andropause Society of Australia Affiliated to The Andropause Society.

Canadian Andropause Society www.andropause.com

Broda Barnes Foundation www.brodabarnes.org The Broda O. Barnes, M.D. Research Foundation, Inc. is a non-profit organization dedicated to education, research and training in the field of thyroid and metabolic balance.

American Academy of AntiAging Medicine www.worldhealth.net

American College for the Advancement of Medicine www.acam.org/

International Society of Andrology www.andrology.org

Jed Diamond www.menalive.com American resource site.

Vavo www.vavo.com/ Lively portal site for the over forty-five's.

The Third Age www.thirdage.com/ More over forty-five's.

Pubmed www.pubmed.co.uk Medical portal site.

WebMD www.my.webmd.com Medical portal site.

The Mens Resource Network www.themenscenter.com Men's issues, resources ... American site.

Mens Stuff www.menstuff.org National men's resource ... Australian site.

Clinics

UK
Gold Cross Medical Centre
20/20 Harley Street
London W1G 9PG
Tel +44 (0)20 8636 8283
Fax +44 (0)20 8636 8292
Info@goldcrossmedical.com
www.goldcrossmedical.com

Europe
Dr. Michael Hansen, EOCCD President
CPH Cardiovascular Clinic
Esplanaden 34,
B Copenhagen
Denmark DK-1263

Prof. Hermann Behre
Institute of Reproductive Medicine
Dieterwegstrasse 39
Halle 06128 Germany
hermann.behre@medizin.uni-halle.de

USA
Dr. J. L. Tenover
Div. of Gerontology and Geriatrics
1821 Clifton Road, NE,
5th Floor-South Wing
30329 Atlanta, GA
jtenove@emery.edu

Dr. Bruce Wilkin
P.O. Box 150455
Ely, NV
89315 United States of America
blwilkin@idsely.com

Eugene Shippen
1124 Old Mill Road
Wyomissing, PA
19610 United States of America
ershippen@aol.com

Jed Diamond
34133 Shimmins Ridge Road
Willits, CA
95490 United States of America
jed@menalive.com

Tom Bader – Pharmacist
3505 Austin Bluffs Parkway
Suite 101, Colorado Spring, CO
80918 United States of America
twbader@aol.com

Canada
Prof. Roland Tremblay
Centre de recherche CHUL
Laval University Hospital Center
2705 boul. Laurier Ste-Foy, Quebec
G1V 4G2 Canada
roland.r.tremblay@crchul.ulaval.ca

Dr. Clement E. Williams
#103–2419 Bellevue Ave.
West Vancouver B.C.
WV 4T4 Canada
2williams@telus.net

Australia
Dr. David Winstone, Brisbane
trewyn@bigpond.com.au

Dr. Adrian Zentner, Melbourne
zentner@netspace.net.au

Well Men Centers, Perth
wellmencenters@quicknet.net.au

India
Andromeda Andrology Center
www.andrology.com

Books

Carruthers, M., *The Western Way of death: Stress, tension and heart disease*. London and New York: Davis-Poynter and Pantheon Books, 1974

Diamond, J., *Surviving Male Menopause: A guide for women and men*. San Francisco: Source Books, 2000

Diamond, J., *Men Alive: Sexuality, health, and longevity for men over 40*. San Francisco: Source Books, 2000

Colborn, T., Dumanoski, D., Myers, J. P., *Our Stolen Future*. London: Abacus, 1997

Nieschlag, E., Behre, H. M., eds. *Testosterone: Action, deficiency, substitution*. Heidelberg: Springer Verlag, 1998

Labs and Tests

UK, Europe, USA, Quest Diagnostics
– special rates via www.AndroScreen.com

Index

gonorrhea 74
Gooren, Prof. Louis 190
Gould, Dr Duncan 147, 190
gout 2
granulomas 84-5
Greece
  Ancient 2-3, 5-6
  male life patterns in 156-7
Greer, Germaine 40, 96-7
growth 66
growth hormone 65
gyms, and exercise 167

hair 47
Hansen, Dr Michael 27, 89, 183, 197
Harris, Frank 137
health, testosterone effects 61
health maintenance 159-60
heart disease 64, 121-2, 158, 207
  testosterone benefits 44-5
  and vasectomy 89-92
Heller, Dr Carl G. 18-20, 102, 131, 180
hepatitis 74
heredity 65-6
High T Male 62, 112, 199
Hinduism 4, 5
Hippocrates 2-3, 6, 73
Hooper, Dr R. xv
hormonal growth promoters 71, 72
hormone profile 99-100
hormone replacement therapy 160-1, 177, 178-9
  see also testosterone replacement therapy
hormones
  and aging 158
  research 13-15
hot flashes 45-6
Hunter, John 9-10
hydrocele 83
hypertension drugs 132
hypogonadism 3, 107-8, 111-12, 198

hypospadias 69-70
hypothalamus 63, 67

IDUT syndrome 21
immune reactions, following
  vasectomy 84, 86
implants, early 10-11
implants (pellets) 17, 20, 21, 88, 101, 105, 106-8, 135, 206
impotence 138-9
imprinting 123-4
India 3-4, 5, 81, 83
Indonesia, testosterone treatment 194
infertility, and tight clothing 78-9
injections
  for erections 134-5
  testosterone 17, 101, 102-3, 206
intermittent claudication 23
International Society for the Study of
  the Aging Male (ISSAM) 192, 201, 211
irritability 37-9

James, Prof. Vivian 22
jaundice 74
Jayle, Dr M.F. 109
Jesell, David 60
Jews, historic medical knowledge 3
jogging 168
joint problems 30, 31, 46-7, 88
Jones, Sir John Harvey 35

Kaufman, Dr Jean 189, 207-8
Kelce, W.R. 72

labetolol 132
Lader, Prof. Malcolm 169
Laqueur, Ernst 16
Lear, Dr M.W. 52
Leifke, Dr 190
Lespinasse, Dr Victor D. 14
Leydig (interstitial) cells 63, 86
libido